T0355094

Rethinking Meditation

Rethinking Meditation

*Buddhist Meditative Practices in
Ancient and Modern Worlds*

David L. McMahan

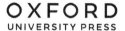
OXFORD
UNIVERSITY PRESS

OXFORD
UNIVERSITY PRESS

Oxford University Press is a department of the University of Oxford. It furthers
the University's objective of excellence in research, scholarship, and education
by publishing worldwide. Oxford is a registered trade mark of Oxford University
Press in the UK and certain other countries.

Published in the United States of America by Oxford University Press
198 Madison Avenue, New York, NY 10016, United States of America.

Library of Congress Cataloging-in-Publication Data
Names: McMahan, David L., author.
Title: Rethinking meditation : Buddhist meditative practices in ancient and modern worlds /
David L. McMahan.
Description: 1. | New York, , NY, United States of America : Oxford University Press, [2023] |
Includes bibliographical references and index.
Identifiers: LCCN 2023007155 (print) | LCCN 2023007156 (ebook) |
ISBN 9780197661741 (c/p) | ISBN 9780197661765 (epub) | ISBN 9780197661772
Subjects: LCSH: Meditation—Buddhism—History. | Mindfulness (Psychology)
Classification: LCC BQ5612 .M36 2023 (print) | LCC BQ5612 (ebook) |
DDC 294.3/4432—dc23/eng/20230222
LC record available at https://lccn.loc.gov/2023007155
LC ebook record available at https://lccn.loc.gov/2023007156

DOI: 10.1093/oso/9780197661741.001.0001

Printed by Sheridan Books, Inc., United States of America

Contents

I. THINKING ABOUT MEDITATION

II. MEDITATION IN CONTEXT

Abbreviations

A	*Anguttara Nikāya*
Aṣṭa	*Aṣṭasāhasrikā Prajñāpāramitā Sūtra*
D	*Dīgha Nikāya*
M	*Majjhima Nikāya*
S	*Saṃyutta Nikāya*
Skt.	*Sanskrit*
SP	*Satipaṭṭhāna Sutta*

Acknowledgments

Two previously published book chapters are reworked and incorporated into this book: "How Meditation Works: Theorizing the Role of Cultural Context in Buddhist Contemplative Practices," in David McMahan and Erik Braun, eds., *Meditation, Buddhism, and Science* (Oxford University Press, 2017); and "Buddhism and Secular Subjectivities: Individualism and Fragmentation in the Mirrors of Secularism," in Richard Payne, ed., *Secularizing Buddhism: New Perspectives on a Dynamic Tradition* (Shambhala, 2021). I thank the publishers for permission to use them.

This book came together with the help of several conferences, grant projects, and individuals. The project was kicked off with a Mind & Life Contemplative Studies Fellowship. I am appreciative of Mind & Life's support as well as their invitations not only to collaborate but also to serve as a gentle critic. Any views, findings, conclusions, or recommendations expressed in this publication do not necessarily reflect those of the Mind & Life Institute.

Other collaborative projects that have fed this work include the putting together of the volume *Meditation, Buddhism, and Science* with Erik Braun. At the time, I saw that volume as a side project, and sometimes I came to think of it as a diversion from completing this book, but the excellent contributors all brought something that helped me think through this work. So thanks to Erik Braun, Julia Cassaniti, Joanna Cook, Bill Edelglass, Bob Sharf, Evan Thompson, Bill Waldron, and Jeff Wilson.

This book has also been enriched by a thoughtful group of international scholars brought together via a grant from the German-Israel Foundation for Scientific Research and Development to research the topic of the ethical foundations of Buddhist meditation. Thanks especially to Eviatar Shulman and Michael Zimmerman for inviting me on board.

The Mangalam Research Center has been part of the incubation of some of the ideas in this work. Thanks to Jack Petranker's indefatigable efforts to bring people together to discuss all things Buddhist, I have benefited from being part of two summer seminars that have proven valuable: "Putting the Buddhism/Science Dialogue on New Footing," funded by the Templeton Foundation, and "The Imagination and Imaginal Worlds in the Mirror of Buddhism," funded by the National Endowment for the Humanities.

Franklin & Marshall College has been a splendid professional home that has given me the freedom to pursue my interests wherever they lead. Thanks especially to my wonderful departmental colleagues, Annette Aronowicz, Stephen Cooper, John Modern, SherAli Tareen, and Rachel Feldman. And to the F&M students I have taught throughout the years, who make several appearances in the book.

Thanks as well to various friends and colleagues who have supported my work in a variety of ways, like inviting me to give talks or contributing chapters that fed into this book, reviewing my manuscripts, writing letters of recommendation for grant proposals, or hanging out in offices, conferences, and bars talking through relevant issues. They include, but I'm certain are not limited to, John Dunne, Ira Helderman, Jonathan Gold, Wendi Adamek, Chuck Prebish, Georges Dreyfus, Justin Brody, Martijn van Beek, Richard Payne, Jay Garfield, Francisca Cho, Hal Roth, Nathan McGovern, David Germano, Greg Johnson, John Harding, Ann Gleig, Linda Heuman, Bernard Faure, Dan Smyer Yü, and members of the Red Rose Sangha (and its offshoots).

Finally, none of this would have meant much without the ridiculously wonderful love and support of partner extraordinaire, Karen Sattler, and son extraordinaire, Caden McMahan.

PART I
THINKING ABOUT MEDITATION

1

Introduction

Dispatches from the Worlds of Meditation: 1a

A young Tibetan Buddhist nun, Sherab Zangmo, enters a pitch-black room for a "dark retreat," in which she meditates in complete darkness for forty-nine days, the same number of days one spends in the *bardo*, the realm in between death and rebirth. During this time, she has a vivid vision of Yeshe Sogyal, an influential eighth-century female Buddhist teacher believed to be the consort of Padmasambhava, who brought Buddhism to Tibet and with whom Sogyal performed *karmamudrā*, meditative sexual yoga. In the vision, the legendary heroine makes three symbolic hand gestures (*mudrās*), after which another historical figure, Yang Gyamtso, the founder of Sherab Zangmo's monastery, also appears. Sherab Zangmo then merges with Yang Gyamtso. "He came to rest on my head and then he dissolved into my body, speech and mind. We became one. I cried and cried. That moment I had a direct experience of the nature of my mind. I have had many experiences, good and bad, but my mind has remained stable, neither good nor bad."[1]

Dispatches from the Worlds of Meditation: 1b

A young woman in a puffy gray dinosaur costume, its head careening and bobbing several feet above her own, walks across Westminster Bridge in London. She is joined by several thousand others who block bridges throughout the city, snarling traffic and carrying signs: "rebel for life"; "fossil fuel era over"; "system change, not climate change." Other actions by the activists, who call themselves Extinction Rebellion, have included a topless protest in which women blockaded Waterloo Bridge with messages written across their bare chests: "climate rape," "climate abuse," and "climate justice"; and another in which men and women in nothing but their underpants stormed Britain's House of Commons during Brexit negotiations, gluing their hands to the glass partition that divides the public from Parliament. Many members of the group are Buddhists or practice Buddhist meditation. At some of their blockades, protestors can be seen sitting cross-legged in meditation posture. Online notices for Extinction Rebellion DC include a meditation and discussion in Malcolm X Park:

Rethinking Meditation. David L. McMahan, Oxford University Press. © Oxford University Press 2023.
DOI: 10.1093/oso/9780197661741.003.0001

"This event is part of an ongoing, peer-led exploration of how we can respond to the climate and ecological emergency with the support of Buddhism, meditation, and other contemplative practices. Our intention is to strengthen our internal and social resources for the challenging work of standing up for a livable and just planet. In recent months, our conversations have focused on the pandemic and racial justice along with the climate crisis. Many of us are members of Extinction Rebellion, a nonviolent international movement demanding action on the climate crisis through non-violent civil disobedience."[2]

Dispatches from the Worlds of Meditation: 1c

A shaven-headed man sits stone-still, legs crossed, back straight, lined up with two dozen others identically clad in black robes on two long, raised platforms in a Zen training monastery in Japan. Another man slowly walks between the two rows of meditators carrying a long wooden stick flattened at the end. He turns to the seated meditator, and they bow slowly to each other, each with his palms pressed together in front of his chest, the meditator bending his head a bit lower than that of the stick-wielder. The meditator remains bent as the other man gently taps his stick on his shoulder, then raises it in the air and smacks the shoulder four times, the staccato cracks echoing sharply through the hall. After he repeats the blows on the other shoulder, they bow solemnly to each other again, and he moves on. Later, on the way to the dining hall, the meditator passes another senior member of monastery and briefly allows his gaze to meet his. The superior punches him in the chest.[3]

Dispatches from the Worlds of Meditation: 1d

A small group saunters into the multipurpose room of a Unitarian church. They are men and women, mostly white, some young but most graying, wearing t-shirts, jeans, sweatpants, and yoga pants. Some bring their own cushions and place them alongside some chairs for those with bad backs. They chat casually until the meditation teacher rings a bell and they take their seats. She welcomes everyone and goes through a brief set of instructions, which most have heard before: straighten the back, relax the body, focus on the breath and count each one silently in cycles of ten; if your attention wanders and you lose count, don't fret about it, just calmly bring it back to the breath and begin the counting again at one. Try to remain in the present moment and not drift to anticipation of the future or rumination about the past. Observe your thoughts or feelings; do not judge them. She rings the bell again, and meditators sit for 25 minutes. Afterward, another participant reads aloud a short chapter from a book on Buddhism written by a well-known contemporary meditation teacher. The group discusses the reading for fifteen minutes or so, then they disassemble the makeshift meditation room, chat a bit more, and make their way home. The next day, the teacher gives the same instructions, purged of any reference to Buddhism, to employees at a midsized tech company.

Meditative Practices, Ancient and Modern

These snapshots of Buddhist and Buddhist-derived meditative practices today represent only a few of the dizzying array that have emerged in the long and culturally diverse history of Buddhism, spanning many cultural and geographic regions and over 2,500 years. Others include practices aimed at transcending the world entirely and existing eternally in a state of disembodied bliss; practices in which meditators imagine external images of a buddha being inhaled through the nostrils, deposited, and arranged in specific places in the body, where they will grow like babies in the womb into a fully awakened buddha within (Crosby 2013); practices involving the detailed visualization of corpses decaying; meditative programs requiring a period of three years and three months isolated in a mountain cave or retreat (Kongtrul 1994); practices involving intricate visualizations of energy-channels, written letters, and deities circulating within the body (Hatchell 2014); practices that require the gathering back of *kwan*, "spirits of the person," that normally inhabit the body but have strayed, causing depression, ill-health, or affliction by malign spirits (Cassiniti 2017).

Yet if you are seeking out meditation today in North America and Europe—and, increasingly, in the rest of the world as well—you will likely encounter one particular type, the one illustrated in the fourth example above, often under the label "mindfulness." There are many places in the United States, where I live, to encounter Buddhist and Buddhist-derived meditative practices under this label: Zen monasteries, Insight Meditation centers, health clubs, colleges, psychologists' offices, corporations, liberal Christian churches, and cardiac rehabilitation centers. If you pursue meditation or mindfulness practices in any of those widely diverse settings, you will likely get the same basic initial instructions and the same concept of what mindfulness is and what it does. One of the most influential formulations is that of one of the pioneers of the contemporary mindfulness movement, Jon Kabat-Zinn. Mindfulness, according to Kabat-Zinn, is "the awareness that arises from paying attention, on purpose, in the present moment, and non-judgmentally" (2013 [1990], lvii). Although the term has a long and diverse history, mindfulness today has come to mean the nonjudgmental awareness of the present moment mentioned above—what I have come to think of as the Standard Version of meditation. There are many variations, but the basic approach is strikingly similar in all of them, whether you are at a YMCA in Salt Lake City or a Buddhist monastery in the Catskills. When I refer to it as the Standard Version, I don't mean it in a derogatory way. I have done it myself and have recommended it to those I think it might benefit from it. But as a historian of religion, I am struck by the way one particular form of meditation has quickly become dominant in so many settings, and I decided it was worthy of historical, cultural, and philosophical investigation.

Indeed, this practice has become ubiquitous across "the West" today and has circulated back to Asia, where, for example, a resident of Tokyo might be more likely to meditate at a mindfulness class in the neighborhood gym than at the local Buddhist temple. Countless articles in popular magazines promote its benefits, often depicting it as a panacea for problems as wide-ranging as anxiety, depression, heart disease, relationship issues, inability to focus, eating disorders, and psoriasis. It is widely used in psychotherapy (Helderman 2019), and there are bestselling books on mindfulness and meditation not only by Buddhist monks but also by medical doctors, psychologists, computer engineers, business consultants, and a US congressman (Tim Ryan (D), Ohio). It is taught in public schools and universities, corporations, hospitals, prisons, and the US military, and is offered by Britain's National Health Service. In North America, several basic forms of Buddhist meditation began gaining traction in the counterculture movements of the mid-to-late twentieth century and more recently have seeped into countless cultural niches, including the most mainstream. In the 1980s, when I first encountered it, it was still a fringe activity, the province of Beat poets, avant-garde musicians, and ageing hippies. Now it is something your family doctor recommends, along with exercising and eating your vegetables.

The way I came to be interested in the subject is a familiar story, nearly an American cliché. I began to explore meditation in my teens in reaction to my growing skepticism of the conservative Christian faith I grew up with. The virgin birth, Christ rising from the dead, the miracles, the atonement, and the stark division between the saved (a vanishingly small number of "true Christians") and the lost (almost everyone outside a few small denominations)—my already enfeebled faith in all of these ideas seemed to reach a tipping point and collapse in the face of the surrounding culture and my education. Far from a crisis, it was liberating to indulge in pleasures that I previously suspected might imperil my immortal soul. But equally exciting was the intellectual space that I felt open up. In a soulless shopping mall bookstore, I gathered several random volumes on Buddhism, Hinduism, "perennial philosophy,"[4] and "mysticism" in an effort to rebuild a coherent worldview. These books informed me that there was a singular Truth at the heart of all major philosophies and religions, and that the road to this Truth was through various meditative practices. This appealed to me, in part, because it promised something other than doctrines to be "believed"; it promised experiential verification shared by centuries of mystics. Meditation, they claimed, was an internal science, as exacting as the various "external" sciences, that would bring meditators to a Truth as certain as the law of gravity.

Two early and profound experiences with meditation convinced me of its value. One occurred while I was in college and studying meditation with a Zen teacher in the lineage of the famous Shunryu Suzuki, Rōshi. I got the hang of it pretty quickly and began a regular practice. One Sunday afternoon, I sat on my bed listening to Steve Reich's *Music for Eighteen Musicians* and fell into a deep state of calm. As the piece ended, I shifted to my makeshift cushion, and the calm became more pervasive as I saw for the first time how many of the things that worried, concerned, and vexed me were creations of my own mind and not fixed impositions of the world upon me. It was profoundly freeing. Later, I went downstairs to the food counter in my building and noticed the other students in line. They all exuded a jittery nervousness and anxiety that I hadn't noticed before, and I wanted to tell them—what, exactly?—that they didn't have to worry so much, that their anxiety was just a trick their minds were playing on them, that everything was alright. Of course, I didn't tell them that, and the next day I dutifully rejoined the jittery, worried masses, but with an insight into how the mind constructs at least some of its own problems. I was newly impressed by the Buddhist analysis of this phenomenon that I was learning about.

The second experience occurred one day a few years later when I was sitting cross-legged on a saggy single bed in my musty one-room apartment. As I sat watching my breath, suddenly the boundaries between myself and the world seemed to disappear, and I perceived myself as something like a bubble in an infinitely vast, all-encompassing, frothing sea of consciousness. Everything I thought I was seemed thoroughly insubstantial, and what little was left threatened to dissipate into the endless plenum. The experience seemed to match perfectly the literature I had been reading on meditation, mysticism, Buddhism, and Hinduism. It was the famous vision of Krishna in the *Bhagavad Gītā*, a cosmic infinity of which I was a part, but to which "I" was utterly insignificant, even illusory. It was at once ecstatic and utterly terrifying. At one point, I felt my heart pounding so rapidly I feared that my body would not be able to survive and, illusory as my ego now seemed, I was not ready to relinquish it. I sent forth a kind of prayer, a plea for help to no one in particular, and the sea suddenly became calm and enveloping, taking on a feminine, maternal, comforting quality.

I tried to capture what I had experienced in writing, and it came out gibberish. For every statement that I wrote, it seemed the opposite was equally true. One sentence wrapped around in a circle to join its own beginning. It seemed inconceivable that I would go back to my ordinary life. "This was the big day," I told a worried friend that evening. After I tried to relate the experience, he asked what I was going to do now. "Just live," I said with the placid confidence of the newly awakened. After a few days, I was no longer "just living," but doing all of the other things college students do: morosely studying for exams, wondering if the woman I was dating was right for me, hanging out with friends.

In many Buddhist traditions, it is considered gauche at best to discuss one's meditative experiences, especially one's "accomplishments." I don't relate them, however, to convince the reader of the meditative prowess of my young self, nor to suggest any particular insight or spiritual development. Just the opposite, in fact. For, while I had felt such assurance in the moment, as the experiences faded and as the years passed, inevitable questions arose that eroded my certainty that I had encountered transcendent truth. If I had been steeped in a study of Christian literature, would I have understood the infinity I encountered as God? Would Jesus have been my savior and comforter rather than the mysterious feminine presence? Was my experience simply the result of an altered consciousness, perhaps some neural misfires, rather than seeing things as they truly are? Was it a bit suspicious that it seemed to confirm the Asian philosophical and religious literature—and its western interpretations—that I had been enthusiastically reading? Was this really an experience that propelled me beyond all of my beliefs, assumptions, and learning, or did it just magnify them?

My exploration of these questions in personal reading, in graduate school, in my academic research as a historian of religion, in my travels in Asia, and in conversations and interviews with meditators, from monks living deep in forest retreats to urban professionals—as well as in my continuing, life-long experiments with meditation—has convinced me that the Perennialist, or "mysticism," explanation of what these practices do is inadequate. Thus, my second loss of faith was in the promise that meditation breaks through to a pristine, unmediated, unambiguous, and universal Truth beyond the "trappings" of particular religions and all culturally informed assumptions, biases, and conditioning—and that all meditative traditions culminate in that Truth. Steeped in universalist assumptions, this view seems incapable of dealing with the questions above, questions ultimately of the relationship between meditative practices and cultural context. Similar questions have been taken up previously by scholars, for example, in a debate between Robert Forman and Steven Katz that revolved around the question of "pure experience." Forman insisted that there is, in fact, a universal mystical experience that transcends all cultural, linguistic, and historical conditioning, while Katz declared that "there are no unmediated experiences" (Katz 1978, Forman 1990). I am not interested in rehashing that debate here, and, in fact, I make no pronouncements on the question, perhaps ultimately unanswerable, of whether experiences that are unmediated by language, concepts, and culture are possible. More modestly, I want to examine how cultural context does impinge on meditative experiences and, along the way, suggest that there is a strong tendency in contemporary discourse on meditation to dismiss such contexts and thereby mistake culturally mediated experiences for achieving a universal view from nowhere. David Germano puts the issue well: "Practitioners, secular adaptors, many scientists, and some humanists often share a dismissive attitude toward culture and context when it comes to the religiously charged question of contemplation, assuming that meditative experience is primarily about extraordinary individual states, so extraordinary that we might identify and extract a particular practice from all its cultural context, and somehow it might come out clean."[5]

And yet, though meditative practices are about more than just "extraordinary individual states," I have no doubt that they have profound effects on individuals, are conducive to novel and valuable personal insights and ethical reflection, and can be truly transformative. So how does meditation work, then? In what follows, I don't attempt anything like a comprehensive answer to that question, but I do want to explore the issue of how culture informs and interacts with meditative practices. My approach focuses less on big, dramatic experiences than on the mundane, everyday work that such practices do in people's lives—lives inevitably embedded in particular cultures and subcultures. It draws upon a variety of philosophical, anthropological, and psychological approaches that examine how people form character, develop capacities and dispositions, cultivate ethical orientations, and come to embody particular modes of being in the world. This inquiry is also inevitably bound up with a genealogical question: how did the particular forms of meditation that have become ubiquitous today—the various forms of the Standard Version—come to be what they are? That is, what are some of the factors by which modern and late-modern cultures created spaces for contemporary Buddhist and Buddhist-derived mindfulness and meditation practices?

Currently, tumultuous "mindfulness wars" perturb the worlds of meditation, and it would be timely and tempting to dive into these debates: to interrogate whether the current mindfulness movement is, on the one hand, a truly revolutionary psychospiritual technology that can transform individuals and societies, a therapy for bringing much-needed peace for frazzled citizens of a frenetically changing world, and a treatment for numerous physical and mental health problems; or, on the other hand, a tool of neoliberal capitalism, a fetishistic distraction from real-world problems, an appropriation of ancient indigenous practices by colonial powers and their descendants, or a dangerous practice that can sometimes lead to psychological harm rather than peace of mind. Much of what I discuss here will have bearing on such issues, but instead of aiming directly at them, I instead want to poke around underneath these questions, to examine some of the assumptions, history, and forms of life on which they rest, to rethink the underlying forces that animate them in the contemporary moment.

I realize that "thinking" about mindfulness and meditation—let alone, "rethinking"—may strike some as an oxymoron. Isn't meditation, after all, about *not* thinking? While it is true that some meditative practices involve cutting off ordinary thought-processes, part of my argument is that this is actually a too-limited way to, well, think about them. And, indeed, rethinking meditation is something that Buddhist philosophers themselves have been doing for centuries in countless volumes on how meditative practices relate to the mind, to ethics, and to the understanding of what human beings are. I do so in a similar spirit.

Filters and Magnets

Consider for a moment how unlikely it is that practices developed by celibate recluses in South Asia over twenty-five centuries ago who renounced their possessions, homes, caste, and family identities to search their minds for a way to transcend sickness, ageing, and death—indeed the entire world—would be adapted to help middle-class professionals function better at work, bond with their families, manage their health, and find calm amid the frantic pace of modern life—even improve their golf game or sex life. How did this happen? The answer to these questions proffered by popular books is simple: meditation works. It is a simple, effective means to calm the mind down, examine it, get beyond impulsive reactions, and allow new insights and possibilities to emerge, making space for distancing oneself from one's own emotional tumult and internal narratives. Today, it is often described as a kind of scientific technique or technological enterprise—a way of "mind hacking." Meditation teachers will sometimes say that what I have called the Standard Version is the foundational meditative practice that the Buddha taught over 2,500 years ago, and which has been transmitted virtually unchanged down through the centuries to us today. The "cultural baggage" surrounding the practices has changed, but the essence is intact, and what it does for people, whether you're a Buddhist monk or a corporate executive, remains the same. These stories, I believe, are misleading. The one I will tell is more complicated; it is one of filters and magnets.

Most of the vast array of meditative practices that have emerged in Buddhist traditions have been filtered out of typical contemporary practice.[6] The filters are generally accepted ideas, tacit notions, and background ideologies prevalent in modernity (let's say, beginning with the European Enlightenment) and late modernity (roughly the second half of the twentieth century to the present) that screen out things that don't make immediate sense in those cultural contexts. For example, the dominant ideas of what human beings are and how they are constituted—we are biological beings whose minds are inseparable from our brains—filters out the likelihood that a long-deceased person might appear above your head, descend into your body, and become one with you for the rest of your days, as in the account above of Sherab Zangmo, the Tibetan nun. What makes it through the filters of modernity are practices that can make intuitive sense and find a home within the categories in which we are accustomed to think, the affective domains in which we habitually feel, the aesthetic sensibilities through which we typically perceive things, and the social, political, and institutional realities within which we are embedded. These filters have allowed only a trickle of meditative practices through to the mainstream of our world. Now, granted, Sherab Zangmo had American and European devotees who revered her and may accept quite literally the extraordinary things she reported. Moreover, contemporary Americans and Europeans have endured years-long meditation retreats in Himalayan caves, month-long retreats in pitch darkness, complex tantric visualizations, and the challenges of rigorous Japanese Zen monastic training. Such things, however, remain on the margins at this point, while the Standard Version has proliferated widely.

In addition to filters, there are magnets that attract certain practices from Buddhist traditions and leave behind others. Elsewhere I have discussed how, for example, ideas in Romanticism, Transcendentalism, scientific rationalism, Christianity, and psychology have magnetically attracted certain features of Buddhism—basic meditation practices, certain ethical and philosophical ideas (McMahan 2008). These ways of thinking and being have drawn forth particular resonant practices from the great diversity of practices in the Buddhist traditions—and not just drawn them forth but transformed and repurposed them. Magnets only pick up things with certain properties, remaining indifferent to the rest. They serve as the conditions of possibility for the growth of these practices outside their native geographic and intellectual homes. For example, as we shall see in chapter 8, Henry David Thoreau and others in nineteenth-century America extolled the value of attentiveness to the natural world and to the mind itself as an antidote to the increasing mechanization of life in the emerging industrial age, with its factories and assembly plants disrupting the agrarian rhythms attuned to the world of plants and animals. Concerns about young people's ability to focus—which, it turns out, were not exclusive to the age of cell phones and social media apps—led to interest in systematic training of the attention in the nineteenth century, creating fertile ground for the introduction of Asian contemplative practices. Nineteenth- and early twentieth-century Buddhists in Japan, Ceylon, and China presented Buddhism as a rational system of philosophy, ethics, and techniques of "scientifically" investigating the mind and world, thus magnetically drawing it to lettered Americans and Europeans disenchanted by "religion" and "superstition." Part of my aim in this book is to provide some examples of such filters and magnets that created the conditions for the development of Buddhist and Buddhist-derived meditative practices as popular practices of self-transformation.

Themes of the Book

Historical and Genealogical Study

I have a few aims in my examination of these practices. First, I want to explore some relevant threads in the historical fabric of Buddhist meditation. This book in no way attempts to be a comprehensive history or survey of the many such practices; rather, it presents a genealogy of some specific elements in classical Buddhist traditions that have fed into contemporary meditative practices—those that have made it through the filters of modernity. It asks: out of the many forms of Buddhist meditation that have developed over two and a half millennia, how and why were particular practices selected to coalesce into the Standard Version today? Part of the answer might be simple historical accident. Certain people from certain traditions had opportunities, for example, to bring their preferred practices to the West, where they happened to encounter people who promoted them, developed them, reconfigured them to contemporary purposes. Such encounters were certainly numerous. But they were not just dictated by random chance. Certain features of the modern world—social and political conditions, scientific developments, literature, historical crises—created a network of conditions, a historical context, that *called forth* particular practices into this context.

This book will help clarify where certain features of the Standard Version come from as well as how they have become reinvented in recent decades. This complicated lineage goes back to accounts of ancient ascetic practices outlined in the early Buddhist scriptures, picks up bits and pieces of later Mahāyāna Buddhist ideas, along with Chinese, Japanese, and Tibetan elements. These then weave their way into the discourses of the Enlightenment and Romanticism, psychology and Existentialism, midcentury countercultures, and, more recently, cognitive science and neuroscience. This coalition of historical forces brought these pursuits together and produced something new—novel interpretations of meditation, what it does, what it is for, and how it works: it reveals the unconscious mind; it unveils laws of nature in the psyche, like a scientist discovering laws of nature in the physical world; it uncovers hidden motivations, desires, thoughts, allowing one to steer them more consciously; it discloses an authentic and natural self, deeper than the one conditioned by one's particular culture and society. None of these interpretations is derived exclusively from Buddhism itself—they emerged as these practices were alloyed with modern discourses. These novel interpretations and adaptations tell us something about the context itself—how we think and feel, what we take for granted, and how we live in our world, and what are our anxieties, fears, and aspirations.

The point is not simply to insist that contemporary forms of Buddhist and Buddhist-derived meditation differ from classical forms or that they are irreconcilable opposites. Rather, I want to show how the Standard Version does, in fact, inherit particular bits of its DNA from ancient accounts of meditation while at the same time reformulating them in novel ways peculiar to modern modes of thinking and feeling, as well as social and political circumstances. I will present various practices as navigating certain binary oppositions, not to suggest that classical versions of meditation always aim at one thing (renunciation or transcendence, for example) and modern versions the opposite (overcoming stress or heightening efficiency at work); rather, the various forms of meditation I address negotiate generative tensions between various possible tendencies: personal and collective, constructive and deconstructive, active and passive, enchanting and disenchanting, modern and ancient.

Theoretical Argument

Individuals, Cultures, and the Underlying Conceptual Architecture of Late Modernity

There is a theoretical and philosophical component to this work interwoven with the historical and genealogical part. It involves a critique—not of contemporary meditation per se, but of how it is conceived in popular and, sometimes, scholarly literature, particularly that coming from the scientific study of meditation. My purpose here is not to complain that more of the vast number of meditative practices from the Buddhist tradition have not made it through the filters, though that might be an implication. Nor am I piling on to the heap of critics assailing contemporary mindfulness as too superficial, corporatized, appropriative, or inauthentic. My critique will overlap with some of these but I am aiming at something a bit more particular: I want to theorize, broadly, the role of culture in meditative practices. I ask the general question, what role does culture play in meditation?—as well as the more specific question: what role has modern, western, secular, and elite-transnational culture played in its constituting its current forms?

These questions might seem strange for some readers. It seems on the surface that meditation would be the ultimate *individual* practice, a decisive turn away from the external world to the internal. Indeed, many popular descriptions insist that meditation gets you in touch with something essential and authentic inside, uncorrupted by society and culture. I will argue that culture is much more important to meditation than is often assumed and that meditation is actually as much a social and cultural practice as a personal one. I present a picture of meditative practices as cultural practices that do particular work in specific cultural contexts rather than seeing them on the (idealized) model of science—a practice of simple observation that discovers universal truths and frees one to act in light of them. Many accounts today see meditation as something that simply has particular effects on the mind, the brain, and the body. Meditation will make you happier, better at your job, calmer, kinder, more socially adept. And there is little doubt that various meditation techniques will have particular effects on neurological and physiological structures. If you relax your muscles and focus on your breath successfully, your blood pressure and cortisol levels will likely decrease, serotonin may increase, and you might feel a sense of calm and well-being. But how these rudimentary psychophysiological phenomena are processed through the intricacies of thought and emotion is deeply interwoven with the specific concepts, expectations, and affective inclinations that are readily available in particular cultural contexts. They cannot be analyzed in a vacuum.

Even when these higher-level processes are short-circuited by the circumventing of discursive thought common in some meditative practices, how the experience gets integrated into your life when you rise from the cushion—its significance to your ethical decisions, the effect it has as you move about during the day, the hope that it inspires for your general emotional state—is deeply shaped by the web of ideas and values surrounding the practice. And this web is supplied by culture, which shapes not only one's default intuitions about how to behave—as a citizen in a democracy, a consumer in a neoliberal economy, or a subject to an emperor in a medieval aristocracy—but also how one exists in various subcultures, including professions, families, churches, and spiritual communities.

Taking a fuller account of the ways such social and cultural factors shape not just meditative experiences themselves but how meditation is integrated into practitioners' lives, complicates another popular assertion: that meditation circumvents "cultural conditioning," allowing meditators to transcend the apparently pernicious influence of society and allow something authentic and uncontaminated to emerge. My argument is not that meditators do not come to genuinely novel, meaningful, and even liberating insights and experiences through their practice—in fact, I think they do. Rather, seeing these insights and experiences as a matter of transcending the influence of society and culture, or of anything outside of the mind itself, oversimplifies the matter. Ironically, the very idea that culture and society are an impediment to the autonomy of the individual is itself derived from modern, post-Enlightenment *culture*. Meditation has, in other words, been adapted to the post-Enlightenment view of the autonomous individual for whom being with others, being in society, and living in concert with social norms is considered a potential imposition on the individual's freedom. Meditation is thus reframed as the ultimate individualistic practice of the singular mind gazing at itself and discerning the truth of things in isolation. It has become tailored to the modern, western concept of the individual as "essentially the proprietor of his own person, owing nothing to society for them" (MacPherson 1962). Part of what this book attempts is to map out some parts of the underlying ideological infrastructure of modern conceptions of selfhood and to show how modern meditation has been tailored to it.

That infrastructure, however, is not fixed. There are different, overlapping and sometimes competing models of selfhood, including the classical liberal understanding of the rational, autonomous self derived from Enlightenment thought; Romantic versions of the self, emphasizing feeling and internal depths; the political self as the possessor of rights and responsibilities; the calculating self of utilitarianism; the psychological self, with unconscious depths and neuroses; the cerebral self, identified with the brain and its functions. Add to this many religious conceptions of selfhood involving souls or, in the case of Buddhism, a fluid, interdependent process that is *not* a self, and this architecture of modern subjectivities may seem complex and cavernous, containing many tunnels, side-closets, and alcoves. Indeed, I resist the notion that the Modern Self is one thing and, instead, suggest that there is a repertoire of possibilities for imagining what a person is, all in creative and sometimes conflictual tension with one another. Part of the story I tell here is how Buddhist meditation has taken up residence in these various spaces, accommodating some, resisting others, and navigating the various tensions between them.

Meditation as a Cultural Practice

Part of the critique will entail questioning a certain popular conception of meditation that I call the "objectivist" interpretation, which views meditation as a kind of technology for obtaining a transparent, objective view of the interior contents of the mind. Such a privileged view is said to secure a lucid vision of a purely interior reality uncontaminated by cultural conditioning and social forces. I caution against this view, which I have come to think of as a "premature universalism" that takes the insights obtained in meditation to be unmediated, transcultural knowledge of the Way Things Are. A parallel premature universalism is manifest in a lot of scientific literature on meditation, which presumes that meditation is primarily something that happens to the brain and central nervous system, which are essentially the same in everyone; therefore, studying what meditators' brains are doing, for example, in an fMRI scan, will tell you "how meditation works." But how meditation works is not just about brains—it is about *the work meditation does* in particular social contexts that meditators inhabit and the repertoire of possibilities, projects, concepts, and moral visions in those contexts.

Still, I resist the conclusion that meditative practice merely reduplicates or amplifies culturally dominant structures of thought and feeling. It does, I think, do this more than is generally acknowledged. But it also has features, inherited from particular Buddhist ideas and practices, that are conducive to dismantling these structures—calling into question accepted truths, interrogating tacit assumptions, reconfiguring affective habits. There is, therefore, a fundamental tension in many Buddhist meditation practices, bequeathed to their modern iterations, between the *constructive* aspects of meditation—the cultivation of attitudes, virtues, ideas, emotions, ways of thinking and being—and the *deconstructive*—the dismantling of all of these. This is a creative tension that allows for multifarious adaptation in the use of meditation, from practices that simply reinforce dominant habits of thinking and feeling to the radical critical interrogation of personal and cultural assumptions. To illustrate this tension, as well as examine the history of the practices that have fed into contemporary meditation, I will delve into selections from classical Indian meditation literature, as well as citing some other relevant examples from Zen and Tibetan Buddhism.

To further anticipate this kind of investigation of the role of culture in meditation, let's think for a moment about the particular cultural world, and its understanding of selfhood, that has helped birth the Standard Version. Practices that have taken root in the modern West have tended to be those that can be made sense of according to the dominant ways that modern westerners understand the self, that is, as an enclosed, private, subjective interior, separate from an external, objective world. Some thinkers have suggested that modern western people have a stronger sense of separation of internal and external, self and other, than those in other cultures (Makari 2015, Taylor 2007, Luhrmann 2020). Here I am not just talking about *theories* of selfhood, but the everyday sense of self. Meditative practices that have been adapted to contemporary affluent cultures have been pressed into the logic of this model of selfhood and to see it as having to do exclusively with interiority. It also takes pains to avoid things that could be called "supernatural," or even more, "superstitious." Thus the Standard Version avoids talk of gods, ghosts, and spirits—"external" forces—and instead focuses on meditation as a means of knowing the mind and its operations. In contrast to, for example, Korean shamans, who will train their minds to listen for messages from deceased ancestors, or evangelical Christians who cultivate the ability to distinguish the voice of God within from other mental chatter (Luhrmann 2012), meditators in this context will train their minds to treat all mental phenomena as "thoughts," all on the same interior plane, so to speak, none more significant than another, all mere events to be observed with detachment and objectivity. And yet they are also encouraged to seek insights within the constant stream of thoughts—insights into personal problems, into how to put together a poem one has been working on, into the fact that all human life is interconnected—or even more nebulously, into the way the swirl of thoughts resonates with the pattern of the succulent on the shelf, which resembles the eddies in the nearby stream and the whirl of galaxies. All of these insights require training in particular ways of looking at one's own mind, as well as previous knowledge, for example, of modern psychology and cosmology. The Standard Version encourages such insights over the hearing of the spirits, cultivating of supernatural powers, or seeking transcendence of the physical world altogether. It requires, therefore, particular cultural understandings of what "thoughts" are (events "inside" the enclosed space of the mind), what one should do to ascertain them, what is their significance, and how one should act in relation to them.

Yet, there is also a countertendency to the interiority of contemporary meditation that we will also explore, particularly in the last chapter: it has also been used as a way to cultivate a sense of the fluidity in the boundaries of the self, to encourage a melding of self and world, to overcome the isolation and alienation of the atomistic individual and develop a porosity of self that encourages profound connection with other people, the natural world, and the cosmos itself. Meditation today is often called upon to navigate the tension between this sense of the enclosed individual, the rational atomistic self of modernity, and this more porous sense of self.

I should add that my critical analysis of the Standard Version is not meant to be a critique of meditators themselves but how many of us today— ordinary practitioners, scientific researchers, scholars—have come to think about and talk about meditation, what it is, what it does, and how it works. I am trying to get at some unexamined assumptions, often drawn from the background ideologies of the modern West, like individualism and certain folk theories of mind. My purpose is not to complain that Buddhist meditation has become "contaminated" with such assumptions, or to insist that some version of "traditional" Buddhism is better, but rather to show that these assumptions are there and render them more distinct so that we can then evaluate them more precisely. This kind of critical examination is itself rooted in modern, western thought but is also informed by Buddhist thought. The Buddhist tradition has reinvented itself many times over and provided radical critiques of even its own cherished doctrines and practices. In this sense, I see my own inquiry as a deployment not only of the methods that constitute the conglomeration of disciplines that that make up Religious Studies—anthropology, sociology, philosophy, history, literary analysis—but also as resonating with certain elements of Buddhist thought itself—indeed, of meditative inquiry.

Meditation and Secularism

It is often said—by some with a derisive snort and others with a satisfied smile—that Buddhist and Buddhist-derived meditation practices have become secularized. This is certainly true in one sense of the word, in that they have been transported beyond the province of Buddhist "religious" institutions and have spread far and wide into public institutions and settings, taken up by schools, governmental bodies, health clubs, corporations, and universities. But this observation carries with it a too-narrow conception of the secular. For now, we need not go into the various ways in which secularism is construed today (I will address the subject further in chapter 8), but a few comments on how conceptions of the secular impinge on the meditation practices we are discussing are in order.

When people refer to the secularization of meditation, the implication often is that the Buddhist bits have been stripped away, leaving the meditation in the realm of the secular, which is conceived as what is left when "religion" is set aside. Yet, a great deal of research on secularism shows that it is not adequately conceived as simply what is left over when religion is segregated—when you set aside unprovable belief and superstition and settle comfortably into rational debate about established facts. The categories of secular and the religious are themselves a historically recent way of dividing up human experience. Secularism is a discourse that creates such divisions conceptually, but it also consists of cultural formations that structure societies and institutions. In popular parlance, it can designate a worldview aligned with science and naturalism and skeptical of institutional religion. Of course, it is a political project as well: the separation of church and state, the setting up of a realm of rational, public political debate and deliberation separate from the more ethereal convictions and passions of religious life. These categories of religious and secular are modern and coconstitutive and do not simply refer to natural, unambiguous species of phenomena. The religious-secular binary is a historically specific way, not just of *classifying* knowledge, subjectivity, meaning, practice, and power—but also of *constituting* it. The discourse of secularism determines what counts as secular, what counts as religious, what is marginalized as superstition or cult, what qualifies as a legitimate exercise of religion and what doesn't. It instills particular disciplines of subjectivity, curates particular beliefs, cultivates sensibilities, and authorizes normative models of behavior, practice, and, indeed, religion. In this sense, ironically, *secularism is not secular*—that is, it is not what it purports to be: a neutral space of rational discourse and practice free from the irrational subjective passions of religion. Rather, it is a discursive tradition, with values, normative practices, attitudes, prohibitions, and metaphysics—much of it still retaining the underlying ideological apparatus of Protestant Christianity. In this sense, secularism—at least in the West—is a kind of post-Protestantism. This is important with regard to our examination of contemporary meditation practices, for they are often modeled on secular forms of knowledge—particularly the secular knowledge par excellence, science—and are often said to secure access to a kind of objective reality within, free from the vagaries of mere beliefs and the impositions of one culture or another. Secularism itself, however, is cultural—and science has its cultures too (Latour 1993).

Contemporary meditation has been significantly shaped not only by its being conceived in secular terms—as a science of mind, a psychological technique, a means of discerning "natural laws" in the psyche—but also by the laws governing secular and religious spaces. Throughout the twentieth century, as Buddhist meditation became more frequently offered to people beyond Buddhist communities, it was increasingly presented as a nonreligious practice, something that required no belief in particular religious ideas or ideals. Meditation and mindfulness were promoted to the world as definitively secular practices by many of its promoters. In their articulation of Vipassana meditation, for example, S. N. Goenka and his followers have often insisted on the nonsectarian and nonreligious character of the practice. An author at an Indian conference on Vipassana put it this way: "[Vipassana] is not a rite or ritual based on blind faith. There is no visualization of any god, goddess or any other object, or verbalization of any *mantra* or *japa*" (Vipassana Research Institute 1995, 11). According to another author it is "a purely scientific technique, a universal culture of mind, which does not subscribe to any sectarian beliefs, dogmas or rituals. It should be universally acceptable, therefore, as an integral part of education" (21). This characterization of meditation as nonreligious and nonsectarian illustrates the broader trend of paring down the complexity of meditation as it is found in the canonical and commentarial texts, often to a single technique like mindfulness of the breath or sensations. This paring down is part of what has enabled Buddhist and Buddhist-derived meditative practices to spread all over the world so quickly and infuse themselves into many areas of life under the banner of the secular. This is not, by the way, solely a matter of "the West" appropriating or adapting something from "the East." This process began in colonial Asia and has, all along, been a complex, mutual creation of Asian and western actors (Braun 2013). Many of the most prominent Asian Buddhists of the twentieth and twenty-first centuries have promulgated basic mindfulness practices to people outside the Buddhist tradition, promoting them as universally beneficial regardless of religious affiliation or lack thereof. Buddhist luminaries like the Fourteenth Dalai Lama (2011), Yongey Mingyur Rinpoche,[7] and Chögyam Trungpa (in his Shambhala program) have all offered programs and approaches to meditation that they themselves have called "secular," and many others have insisted that basic Buddhist meditation practices can and should be taken into multiple spheres of secular life, from business to law to education to medicine. Perhaps the apex of this effort has been Jon Kabat-Zinn's Mindfulness-Based Stress Reduction (MBSR), which was quite deliberately stripped of religious language and references to Buddhism, even though it was derived from Zen and Vipassana traditions. This has allowed MBSR to be taught and practiced in public schools and government institutions, and the plethora of scientific studies on the effects of various secularized forms of meditation and mindfulness have given them a legitimacy that could only be conferred by its occupation of secular spaces. MBSR and other secular mindfulness practices have also been tailored to the contours of American laws on the separation of church and state. This is an example of how the cultural, political, and legal contexts in which these practices occur shape the practices themselves, along with how their purposes are conceived.

If Buddhist meditation came to Europe and North America on the back of secularism and naturalism, it, like many colonial imports, has never been thoroughly contained by these paradigms. Today we are assured in countless articles and books that meditation is sanctioned by secular authorities and demonstrated effective by scientists, all in the language of a world purged of the supernatural or superstitious. Yet secularity is still haunted by ghosts that have never been completely exorcised from the machine. Scientists may claim that meditation "works" for countless worldly goals, but many practitioners use meditation to assure themselves that there is "more than this," more than the desacralized world portrayed by science. The "more," however, is often sought *within* the "this"—in deeper resonances, dimensions, and aesthetics of the here and now, rather than the *more* of another world in the future—the Pure Land or nirvana. It is a "more" that affirms this-worldliness but at the same time attempts to break open secularism and show that this world exceeds what it seems to be on first glance: the frog plopping in the pond, the chopping of wood, the carrying of water—simple things that are, to contemplative probing, *more*. So the Standard Version isn't simply "secular," in the popular sense of the word denoting strict adherence to a naturalistic or materialistic worldview, despite assurances from mindfulness teachers in public schools or at Goldman Sachs. Rather, it occupies a field of tension between, on the one hand, comfort in the dominant discourse of secularity—the naturalistic worldview taught in public schools and taken for granted in mainstream newspapers, the established normativities of late modernity—and, on the other hand, the destabilization of that very discourse, and the bending of it toward the possibility of a kind of secular re-enchantment of the world.

Ethical Subjects

The later sections of the book move on from the argument that meditation is a cultural activity to the question of *how* meditation has been reconfigured in the conditions of late modernity and become nestled in the cultural values of contemporary secularism and liberalism.[8] Despite the emergence of a Standard Version, there is now an unprecedented profusion of uses to which meditative practices are put. My purpose is not to catalog these multifarious deployments but rather to examine some underlying ideals running through many of them—orientations that are built-in to the subterranean conceptual architecture of contemporary social imaginaries.[9] I don't intend to map out the entirety of this underlying architecture but to look at selected parts, examining how contemporary meditation has become refracted through the lens of certain concepts: appreciation, authenticity, autonomy, and interdependence. These are modern concepts, though some have antique roots. They are important enough that I see each as an "ethic" in a particular sense; that is, they are constellations of concepts, values, and ideals through which contemporary meditators interpret self and world, but also that carry implicit directives about how to act in the world. They are not "ethics" in that they are well thought-out positions, at least not for everyone. Rather they are part of the background landscape of ideals and values prevalent in late-modern liberal democracies.

What I call the Ethic of Appreciation highlights the fact that contemporary meditation is far less focused on transcendence of the world than on appreciation of life in all of its diversity, complexity, and nuance. Classical Buddhist texts insist that the body, the material realities of the world, the processes of birth and death, the eating of food, the performing of one's work, and sensual pleasures are all marked by dissatisfaction, ephemerality, and insubstantiality. The imperative in these texts is to break habitual attachments to them, even to develop revulsion for them, and ultimately, to transcend them completely. Contemporary meditators, in contrast, are guided by an implicit injunction to appreciate their lives as embodied beings in a material world and to use their practice to enhance this appreciation. They are encouraged to cherish the beauty of nature, the tastes and textures of food, the sensual delights of a massage or even sex. Failing to do so would be missing the wonder and mystery of existence in the world. Such invitations have roots in the European Enlightenment, Romanticism, and Transcendentalism, humanism, and psychology, with their relative de-emphasis on the supermundane and the affirmation of the value—in some cases, even the sacredness—of this world and of finding transcendence in immanence. But they also reflect broad, historical movements in Buddhist thought, some of which began to question the distinction between nirvana and *saṃsāra*, offering more this-worldly interpretations of awakening and affirming transcendence in immanence, especially in East Asian contexts.

The Ethic of Authenticity and the Ethic of Autonomy are closely related values that wrap Buddhist meditation into the individualistic ethos of modernity. While originally Buddhist meditation was directed toward freedom from the world itself, today freedom can hardly be thought without reference to liberal ideas that have emerged in the last few centuries: freedom of thought, freedom from tyranny, freedom of expression, freedom from oppression, freedom to shape one's own life and destiny, freedom from enslavement to the passions (in favor of reason). It is not that these aspirations are either uniquely modern or completely absent from earlier conceptions of freedom; but the inherited ideas of personal autonomy and freedom are so stitched into the fabric of modern life that they are taken for granted, at least in liberal democratic societies. Contemporary iterations of meditation, therefore, have inevitably been threaded into this fabric as well, repurposed as techniques for the formation of subjects in search of freedom in these distinctive senses.

The concern with navigating freedom and bondage through meditation today often emerges in this language of "social conditioning" versus internal freedom, autonomy versus following "tradition," "authenticity" versus conformity to external norms. The drama of liberation of the individual from external tyranny is transposed into a battle between socially conditioned habits of mind and something authentic within—something original, self-determined, or experientially verified. One becomes the author of one's own life by escaping the internalized dictates of a sick society and pursuing one's own unique, authentic path.

There is something almost inevitable about this way of thinking today, and no doubt, nearly everyone in liberal democratic societies embraces certain aspects of it. We teach our children to think for themselves, to choose their own careers, to find their own paths, to have original thoughts, to avoid simply following the herd. Yet we also know from mountains of evidence in the humanities, social sciences, and psychology that we are fundamentally social creatures who seek out the authentication, justification, and recognition of our peers, and that even our most distinctive artists and writers are taking a plethora of materials from their culture and making something new from it. Moreover, the ideal of a self-authenticating, transparent insight into the workings of one's own mind in beings so vulnerable to cognitive distortions, propaganda, advertising, and so on, can often be a mirage. Social thought has problematized the value of what some have considered an excessively individualistic bent to the discourses of autonomy and authenticity. Thus, I will discuss some contemporary articulations of the kinds of freedom and authenticity that meditation supposedly confers, especially notions of freedom resembling Enlightenment-influenced ideas of the autonomous subject floating freely above social conditions, nestled in a mindful inner citadel, invulnerable to "external" disturbances. If such concepts of internal freedom are inadequate, what kind of freedom might meditative practices offer, then? While not dismissing entirely the "inner citadel" model, I argue, drawing from certain feminist, anthropological, and psychological research, that such practices create possibilities for greater "situated autonomy," a concept that acknowledges the embeddedness of subjects in a nexus of social conditions and in which these practices provide for the expansion of agency through the increased awareness of possibilities for action (i.e., affordances). I also touch on how such conceptions of situated autonomy, as well as the aforementioned deconstructive aspects of meditation, have been important to the development of the recent idea of deploying meditative practices in service of sociopolitical freedom and justice, for example, the dismantling of racist and consumerist habits of mind.

If the ethics of authenticity and autonomy are reliant on a kind of centripetal force that tends toward interiority, in some cases exacerbating the sense of the isolated, autonomous self of the modern West, there are also centrifugal forces in contemporary interpretations of meditation—those that encourage a dissolution of the boundaries between self and world or that call for ethical and political engagement. These often employ what I term the Ethic of Interdependence. This ethic draws more explicitly from Buddhist doctrine, refracted through contemporary conditions, and reinterprets the often fragmented chaos of late modernity as the capacious connectedness of all things. It also carries a rationale for braiding meditative endeavors together with ethical and social responsibility: meditation under this concept cultivates a sense of the porosity of the boundaries between the self and other and emphasizes the systematicity (rather than the individuality) of suffering and the responsibility to care for others and for the planet, again, in contrast to an exclusive focus on meditation as the cultivation of personal peace of mind.

I don't claim that these particular four "ethics" constituting parts of the underlying architecture of secularism are the only such components relevant to contemporary meditation, but I believe they are important ones. In fact, there are others that are more obvious than these, such as what we might call the *ethic of health and well-being* and the *ethic of productivity*. My reason for not focusing more explicitly on these is not that they are unimportant but that others have addressed them ably and thoughtfully.[10] More generally, this book in no way attempts to nail down a definitive understanding of meditation, nor account for all of the ways it might help, transform, or even harm people. It instead attempts to illuminate cross-pressures, tensions, and intersections entailed in meditative practices today in order to show that meditation—itself by no means one thing—does not simply *do* one thing. It might activate opposing tendencies within a society and even within the same practitioner: activity and passivity, agitation and serenity, acceptance and political urgency, self-containment and interconnection.

Finally, I have attempted to make this book a bit more accessible to nonspecialists than academic books tend to be, avoiding too much reliance on discipline-specific jargon and avoiding long digressions into technical and theoretical issues. This might disappoint my fellow scholars of religion, but it is because my intended audience is not only them but also scholars in other fields who now study meditation—psychologists, neuroscientists, and philosophers—as well as nonacademic practitioners of meditation. For it is the ideas about meditation that often circulate among scientists and practitioners, more than scholars of the humanities, that I want to scrutinize and, in some cases, rethink. Those hoping for methodological consistency and theoretical tidiness will also be disappointed. I roam rather promiscuously among anthropological, philosophical, psychological, and historical methodologies and theoretical frameworks. I both critique and draw from ideas in the cognitive sciences. I employ a mixture of a hermeneutics of suspicion and sympathy. I perform my research as an outsider, but I have also studied with meditation teachers, been part of meditation groups, and done some form of meditative practice for the majority of my adult days. I am not doing "Buddhist theology"—that is, thinking from an explicitly Buddhist position—and some of my conclusions might be at odds with Buddhist (as well as secular mindfulness) orthodoxies; yet, I am also sympathetic to much in Buddhist thought, practice, and ethics and feel little obligation to insulate myself from its influence on my thinking. I think *about* Buddhism and, also, *along with* Buddhism—and sometimes, against it.

This book also reflects my particular scholarly idiosyncrasies. I began my career as a specialist in Indian Buddhism, working with Sanskrit texts like the Perfection of Wisdom (*prajñāpāramitā*) literature and the *Gaṇḍavyūha Sūtra*, along with the early Buddhist discourses in the canonical language of Pali. As a side project, I began exploring the emergence of modern, transnational forms of Buddhism, and this project snowballed into a major part of my research. This book brings together these two poles, exploring uniquely modern and contemporary articulations of Buddhist meditation and looking for some of their precedents in classical Indian literature and, to a lesser extent, in the Chan/Zen and Tibetan traditions (in which I have less linguistic competence).

Another scholar with other interests and specializations might tell a different story, for example, with more attention to the significant influence of Tibetan traditions on contemporary versions of Buddhist meditation. Mine follows particular threads among many in the vast and complex tapestry of Buddhist meditative practices. There are many other stories to tell.

2

Neural Maps and Enlightenment Machines

The Enlightenment Machine

Vince Horn and Daniel Rizzuto are excited about the possibility of an Enlightenment Machine. In a conversation recorded on Horn's *Buddhist Geeks* podcast, they muse about the feasibility of a neurofeedback machine that might track one's progress toward enlightenment.[1] Rizzuto is an accomplished neuroscientist, a former Director of Cognitive Neuromodulation at the Computational Memory Lab at the University of Pennsylvania and now the founder and CEO of NIA Therapeutics, which develops brain-stimulating devices for treating memory loss—in other words, not a guy in his parents' basement thinking up cool machines after smoking a joint and casually roaming New Age websites. He and Horn speculate about "neural maps of meditative cartographies," as well as a machine that could assess "where you [are] on the map" during your meditation, thereby possibly "accelerating the process" toward advanced meditative states and even enlightenment itself. This would amount to an attempt to obtain, they say, "empirical data" and an "objective assessment" of "where you're at" in your practice. They agree on the importance of ethical training as a part of the process; might such maps of biological correlates of internal states track the biological foundations of ethical progress? Such objective measures could also help, Rizzuto suggests, with adjudicating "claims" by teachers, presumably to some sort of enlightenment or advanced spiritual status. (Might there be some kind of neural certificate analogous to the *inka* common among recipients of *dharma*-transmission in Zen? A ritually sanctified MRI scan?) Horn ponders the possibility of the Enlightenment Machine sending its data back to a central database that could be used by others to help them chart their neural course through the different

Rethinking Meditation. David L. McMahan, Oxford University Press. © Oxford University Press 2023.
DOI: 10.1093/oso/9780197661741.003.0002

stages of enlightenment. Both Horn and Rizzuto are cautious about such ideas and recognize that tracing out the Eightfold Path in neural pathways is a highly speculative and somewhat playful matter, but they clearly see it as a theoretical possibility.

They are not alone. Andrew Newberg, a neuroscientist at the University of Pennsylvania, along with coauthor Mark Robert Waldman, published a book titled *How Enlightenment Changes Your Brain: The New Science of Transformation* (2016). The book doesn't promise an Enlightenment Machine, but develops the underlying premise that one can, through various neurological measurements, chart a course to enlightenment. It endeavors to provide a

> new model of human awareness, a "spectrum" that begins with instinctual awareness and ends with the experience of Enlightenment. As we progress along this spectrum, we are actually moving from a minimal amount of awareness about the world toward a complete awareness of the whole universe. This map combines ancient wisdom and modern science in ways that make it easy to identify where you are on your path and quest for Enlightenment. (Newberg and Waldman 2016, 1)

Readers who think that the prospect of an Enlightenment Machine is absurd should note that several neural feedback meditation machines are already on the market, albeit with less ambitious goals than those we've mentioned. Muse, The Brain Sensing Headband, whose slogan is "get a better brain in 3 minutes a day," promises that users will "experience the benefits of meditation—without the uncertainty." The device is essentially a portable EEG sensor that fits on the head and "measures your brain activity and gives you real-time feedback on your brain state to help guide your meditation practice."[2] A newer version, Muse 2, also monitors the heart, breath, and posture and sells for $249.99. Of course, meditation apps are currently all the rage. They offer guided meditations straight to your earbuds from your phone and feature soft music and soothing voices giving step-by-step directions. One of the most successful, Headspace, is a multi-billion-dollar company (Widdicombe 2015). But Muse goes a bit further in that it monitors brain waves, thus purporting to confer "objective" information to the practitioner, offering the benefits "without the uncertainty."

Dispatches from the Worlds of Meditation: 2a

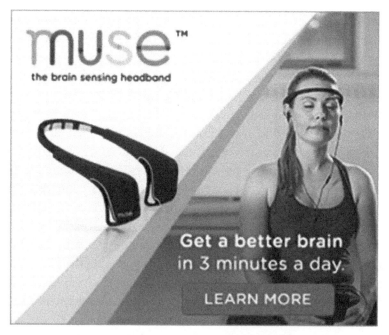

FIGURE 2.1 Muse™ EEG-powered meditation and sleep headband.

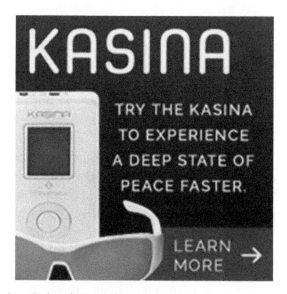

FIGURE 2.2 Kasina Mind Media System.

It is easy either to get seduced by such machinery and its promises of objectivity, certainty, and an electronic shortcut to the peace of mind cultivated by ancient sages—or to dismiss them as high-tech snake oil. Scholars of humanities like myself (as well as some neuroscientists and serious meditators I've spoken with) tend to go the snake oil route. But my purpose here is not to evaluate the efficacy of such devices but rather to examine this language of "certainty" and "objectivity" surrounding them, what assumptions about the mind and knowledge are built into such language, and how such language contributes to a widely promoted notion of how meditation works. In short, a pervasive idea, especially in the scientific study of meditation and popular works piggybacking on this research, is that meditation is, in part, about (1) gaining an objective view of the subjective contents of experience and (2) getting the brain into a specific state that is repeatable, testable, and observable through various neuroimaging and measuring machines. A similar language pervades Horn's and Rizzuto's conversation about the Enlightenment Machine. The machine, they suggest, might give practitioners objective, empirical data that could help practitioners more easily navigate their way not only to calm and focus but also to enlightenment itself. And such measurements could be combined with internal experience, collating both first-person and third-person maps to higher consciousness.

Let's think about some of the presuppositions involved in such speculation—about what kind of implicit ideas form the ground for suggesting that such maps and machines are even theoretically possible—and how these presuppositions infuse modern conceptions of, research on, and even practice of meditation. These presuppositions amount to certain implicit pictures of the human being (anthropologies, in the broad sense of the study of what human beings are), along with associated views of how humans come to know things (epistemologies). These pictures matter to the current research and discussion about Buddhist and Buddhist-derived meditation and mindfulness practices because they not only shape how we think about meditative practices today but also shape the practices themselves. And though they appear to be the taken-for-granted background of much knowledge today, they are contestable—one might even say, metaphysical—pictures. They are the canvas on which scientific truths are painted rather than settled scientific truths themselves.

The pictures I am referring to are (1) a picture of the mind as a container of contents—thoughts, ideas, representations, emotions, etc.—that can be observed through introspection, and (2) a picture of self or personhood as identical with the brain; what some thinkers have called the "cerebral subject" or the "neurochemical self" (Vidal and Ortega 2017, Rose and Abi-Rached 2013). These pictures are such an integral part of the landscape of modern thought that they are not always visible. When they show up, they don't always amount to well-thought-out theoretical positions so much as background assumptions. Philosophical work has addressed them, often quite critically, but modern meditation movements and their neuroscientific study has yet to grapple with them seriously. I don't intend to offer any kind of thorough-going critique of these pictures; rather, I want, first, to point out a couple of ways in which they enter into scientific research as well as popular thinking on mindfulness; second, to offer a few critiques of these ways; and third, to offer a preliminary sketch of an alternative way of thinking about mindfulness and meditative practice, as culturally embedded practices, that will be developed in later chapters. But first, it is worthwhile to look briefly at how we came to speak so often of meditation, objectivity, and science in the same breath.

Meditation as a Science of Mind

The association between Buddhism and science began in the late nineteenth century, in part, as a defensive move by Buddhist reformers in several Asian countries against colonialism, European economic and military hegemony, missionization, and general denigration of the culture and religion of the colonized. Buddhist reformers from Ceylon, China, Japan, and Burma began to frame Buddhism, with its emphasis on causality, absence of a creator god, lack of a doctrine of a nonmaterial soul, and friendliness to the notion of the continuity between humans and animals, as the religion most compatible with modern science. For example, at the World's Parliament of Religions held in Chicago in 1893, the influential Buddhist apologist from Ceylon, Anagarika Dharmapala, characterized Buddhism as accepting the "doctrine of evolution as the only true one, with its corollary, the law of cause and effect," thus allying Buddhism with the cutting-edge scientific revolution of the time, Darwin's theory of evolution (Dharmapala 1965, 9). Likewise, he articulated the Buddhist doctrine of dependent origination—the arising of all phenomena through multiple causes and conditions (including karma)—as being in accord with modern scientific notions of causality, in contrast to the divine action of God. In a similar vein, Paul Carus (1852–1919), an early American enthusiast and popularizer of Buddhism, insisted that Buddhism was the foremost representative of the "religion of science" that would emerge in the modern age: "Buddhism is a religion which knows of no supernatural revelation, and proclaims doctrines that require no other argument than 'come and see'. The Buddha bases his religion solely on man's knowledge of the nature of things, on provable truth" (1915: xiii). This interpretation began to achieve momentum in the late nineteenth and early twentieth centuries, attracting

British and American intellectuals who helped popularize it among the intelligentsia.

Asian Buddhists promoting Buddhism on the global stage and revitalizing it in their own countries also attempted to ally Buddhism with science. Japanese Zen teacher Soyen Shaku, for example, wrote in 1913 that, in his views of causality and other matters, "Buddha's teachings are in exact agreement with the doctrines of modern science" (1993 [1913], 122). Such declarations appealed to educated, liberal Victorian-era Americans and Europeans, some of whom had become disillusioned by Christianity and longed for a religion compatible with current scientific thinking. This articulation of Buddhism also allowed Asian Buddhists to turn the colonial narrative on its head: rather than Europeans bringing civilization, rationality, science, and Christianity to benighted, superstitious Asia, the Buddha had discovered, centuries ago, some of the principles of modern science and, moreover, had promoted a humanistic ethic not reliant on a personal god, miracles, or a special revelation (Lopez 2008, McMahan 2008). This early interpretation of Buddhism as consistent with modern science was, in fact, a selective interpretation, already reshaped for the modern world. Classical Buddhist literature is replete with supernatural beings, miracles, rebirth, and an ancient cosmology with heavens and hells— all conceptions that would be difficult to square with modern scientific concepts. In Buddhist cultures we find ample worship of divine beings, use of talismans, astrology, and rites for the appeasement of demons. The modernized representation of Buddhism as compatible with science emphasized its philosophical and ethical elements, reframing them in accordance with modern thought, while largely ignoring these other elements.

This linking of Buddhism and science set the stage for a more explicit construal of Buddhist meditation as a sort of inner science. As early as the 1930s, the Ceylonese author Soma Thera described "the Way of Mindfulness" as "the objective way of viewing anything whatsoever." "This 'objective' way of looking at a thing, freed from considerations of the personal reactions to that thing, is the pith of the method and constitutes what is called 'knowing as it is' (*yathabhuta ñanadassana*)."[3] This emphasis on "objectivity" invoked another key term in scientific terminology, just as the previous generation of Buddhist reformers had emphasized causality and evolution. The influential German-born Theravada monk Nyanaponika Thera (born Siegmund Feniger, 1901–1994) wrote in 1954 of meditative attention as being a kind of scientific attitude of "unprejudiced receptivity" to things, "bare attention," reduction of the subjective element in judgment, and "deferring judgment until a careful examination of the facts has been made." This, he claimed, is the "genuine spirit of the research worker" (Nyanaponika 1954, 42). The influential Vipassanā teacher, S. N. Goenka (1924–2013), often claimed that Vipassanā, a modern reformulation of early Buddhist meditation practices, "is beyond all religion, beyond all sects, beyond all beliefs, beyond all dogmas and cults—it is a pure science of mind and matter" (2002, 14). Vipassanā, he frequently insisted, was not a religious practice, but a scientific endeavor that discovered the *dharma*—not in the sense of the Buddha's doctrine but, rather, the universal way things are, the natural order of things as manifested in the mind and discovered in unbiased introspective observation (Stuart 2020). A contemporary disciple of Goenka describes the Buddha as a "super-scientist" whose meditative experiments allowed him to "understand how his physical and mental structure functioned. His experiment was scientific in the sense that his goal was to understand objective facts of nature which exist independently of his observing them, through a process of systematic observation which was distorted by his own subjectivity as little as possible."[4] In a similar vein, Alan Wallace has characterized advanced meditators as akin to scientific researchers performing repeatable experiments, making "discoveries . . . based on firsthand experience," then subjecting them to "peer review by their fellow contemplatives, who may debate the merits or defects of the reported findings" (2003, 9). And when Sam Harris refers to Buddhism "without the unjustified bits" as "essentially a first-person science," he is boiling the entire tradition down to the contemporary Standard Version of mindfulness, which he considers to be a scientific technique for observing the mind (2014, 209). Today the characterization of meditation as a kind of empirical investigation of the contents of consciousness, fundamental laws of the mind, or one's true and authentic nature, have come to permeate mindfulness and meditation literature. An interviewee in Joanna Cook's fieldwork with practitioners of mindfulness-based cognitive therapy (MBCT) therapist-training program at Exeter University distills the idea succinctly:

> Science creates protocols to more clearly understand an empirically verifiable world. We can do that internally too. The Buddhists have been doing this for over 2,500 years and have replicated the same insights over and over and over through thousands and thousands of people. Ok, that's a subjective experience, but that's a shared experience, no less valid than the objectivity of ordinary science. (Cook 2017, 114–15)

From this history of framing meditation as a kind of internal science, it was not a large leap to examining it as an *object* of scientific investigation. In 1992, scientists from the United States lugged heavy equipment up the side of a Himalayan mountain above Dharamsala, India, to hook up Tibetan yogis living in caves to electroencephalography (EEG) devices— instruments that record electric activity in the brain— along with various other imaging devices. It was one of the opening volleys in the recent wave of neuroscientific studies that have attempted to unlock the secrets of the meditative mind (a previous wave began in the 1960s and focused mainly on Transcendental Meditation). For centuries Buddhist monks have gone into small mountain caves and tiny forest huts to meditate, sometimes for years at a stretch. Only recently, however, have they wedged their way into the cramped quarters of functional magnetic resonance imagery (fMRI) machines in research hubs like the Center for Healthy Minds at the University of Wisconsin-Madison. These machines measure blood flow in various parts of the brain in real time, thus indicating heightened activity, and have become an important component in studies of the effects of meditative practices on the body and mind.

Such studies, along with other kinds of clinical trials, have exploded in the last three decades. Publications on "mindfulness" in scientific journals have increased from a total of 13 in the entire decade of the 1980s to 92 in the 1990s to 1,203 in the year 2019.[5] Researchers have studied the effects of meditation on perception, attention, anxiety, regulation of emotional states, responses to stressful stimuli, immune system functioning, and central nervous system activity. Scientists have measured the degree to which meditation produces brainwaves associated with various states of concentration, relaxation, and emotional well-being. They have measured how it affects blood flow in various areas of the brain associated with different cognitive functions such as attentiveness and the processing of sensory information. Some scientists have used meditation studies to help them understand neuroplasticity—the ability of the brain to generate new cells and neural connections—and have asserted that the brain changes measurably as a result of regular and prolonged meditation. Researchers have found evidence that some forms of meditation may improve immune function, help reverse heart disease, reduce chronic pain, decrease depression and anxiety, and suppress the overproduction of stress hormones. Scientists have studied the effects of some practices on neural activity in regions of the brain they claim are associated with happiness and well-being and the diminishing of emotions like hatred and anger.[6]

Much of this research has been done on basic mindfulness practices, versions of the Standard Version. Some, however, has involved meditations on loving-kindness, and a few experiments have been performed on more esoteric Tibetan practices such as *tummo*, the generation of internal heat, which appears to create a sustained rise in body temperature through a combination of visualization and muscular movements. Much of this research has been carried out in the most prestigious academic institutions in North America and Europe, including Harvard, Stanford, and Oxford universities. Nevertheless, many of these experiments have been on small populations, questions have been raised about methodology, and reviews of the research find that still more needs to be done to establish firmly what are currently somewhat tentative conclusions (Ospina et al. 2007, Tang et al. 2015).

It is this research that has ushered Buddhist and Buddhist-derived meditation practices from the realm of the exotic and esoteric into the mainstream in a few short decades. It combines legitimacy derived from scientific attention with the allure of ancient wisdom revived to alleviate the ills of modernity. Popular media has eagerly followed the scientific research on meditation, often exaggerating its findings and elevating mindfulness to a panacea for virtually any physical or mental problem (Heuman 2014). Popular books and articles have proliferated promising that mindfulness can not only alleviate physical and psychological ailments but also enhance performance, productivity, and enjoyment of a nearly endless array of activities from playing tennis to working at the office to making love. Thus, entirely new cultures of meditation have proliferated not only outside the monastic institutions, where they have been nearly exclusively housed for centuries, but outside any remaining doctrinal influence from the Buddhist traditions in which they emerged. These cultures—fitness, corporate, military, academic, and many others—create their own meanings of and purposes for meditation (Wilson 2014). Yet they all to some extent stake the legitimacy of the practice on its claim to have been tested and verified scientifically. Pick up any popular book on meditation or mindfulness and you will likely see claims to scientific validation in the first couple pages.

The Theater-of-the-Mind Model of Mindfulness

Scientific studies, of course, need to operationalize: that is, they need to define how a phenomenon is observed, measured, and manipulated. The phenomenon measured needs to be isolated from other phenomena that might muddle the data. And studies must be repeatable, thus definitions must be standardized so different researchers know that they are examining the same thing in different studies. Thus, despite critiques that "mindfulness" has been rather vaguely defined across scientific studies, a general concept has emerged that has become quite standardized in both scientific and popular literature, at least when compared to the rich array of practices in the Buddhist traditions from which they have been extracted. Again, this is what I call the Standard Version. Psychologist Scott Bishop offers a definition that has been used in a great deal of clinical research: mindfulness is "a kind of nonelaborative, nonjudgmental, present-centered awareness in which each thought, feeling, or sensation that arises in the attentional field is acknowledged and accepted as it is" (Bishop et al. 2004).

This definition draws to some extent on Buddhist meditation practices, but it also contains echoes of a particular model of the mind and its activities that has been dominant in modern western thought since Descartes—the representational model, or what has more recently been dubbed the "theater of the mind" epistemic model. Although many philosophers today are highly critical of this model, it still holds sway in popular conceptions of how the mind knows things and is still influential in some cognitive science and neuroscience research. It suggests that the mind cannot directly know objects, but only their representations in the mind. Science, with its methods of empirical observation and reasoned analysis, can help us coordinate the representations in the mind with the external world. This model takes as its ideal that our most accurate access to things is brought about through disengaged observation, quelling of emotions, and neutralization of any particular social or cultural perspective in order that the disengaged, independent subject may encounter things as they are from a presuppositionless neutrality. The individual subject has a clear, privileged, and private view of these interior contents of consciousness. The mind is like a container with private contents of experience, a personal theater with representations projected onto a screen of which the individual is a spectator. When the internal representations match the external, mind-independent reality, one achieves truth.

Under the tacit influence of this model, meditation becomes a kind of refined method of observing interior states and ascertaining them with the same kind of (idealized) objective clarity as objects of scientific investigation. Rather than observing external objects, one observes internal representations themselves, often referred to in modern meditation literature as "thoughts." Setting aside "judgments," which presumably distort our primary access to these mental phenomena as they are, implicitly allows immediate, unbiased, and clear access to those phenomena. Thus, modern iterations of mindfulness have been crafted to resemble the kind of neutrality to which the secular, scientific gaze rooted in European Enlightenment epistemology aspires: a nonjudgmental, nonemotional observation free of bias, sectarian influence, religion, and superstition.

With this picture in mind, notice how modern mindfulness literature suggests that mindfulness is a kind of interior science by presenting it as the unbiased, nonjudgmental observation of the contents of consciousness with clarity and distinction; that is, one sees, through introspection, the primary "data" of consciousness "as it is," rather than getting caught in socially and culturally conditioned concepts, value-judgments, ruminations, emotional reactions, and mind-wandering that normally distort this primary data. On this model of mindfulness, one can, upon accessing this primary data, choose what desires, impulses, and ideas to actualize, rather than being mechanically pulled by impulse. It's not that this model implies that meditation is value-free and devoid of ethical content; a lot of mindfulness literature has at least implied values and ethical orientations. Rather, it's that the initial experience of the observation of mind, the initial mindful contact with the stream of consciousness, is free of judgment, values, and conditioning. Then, having had this initial experience of thoughts and feelings as they are, one is freer to decide what to do with them. Mindfulness is often presented as a matter of having the freedom to "choose" one's states of mind or at least which states on which to act. One steps back, observes without reacting, then is able to circumvent impulsive responses, and in doing so open up a space for choosing one's response based on reflection on one's intentions and ethical values.

Dispatches from the Worlds of Meditation: 2b

You are the Subject and everything else is an object of your knowledge, perception, or awareness, and therefore not you. What it means is that as the Subject, you are ultimately responsible for how you respond to everything you experience. Although some people may try, no one can dictate your response to any person, situation, or event, or anything else that you experience. It's up to you, every time, because it is your mind that determines your interpretation or perception of it, which drives your response to it.

—Elisabeth Thornton, *The Objective Leader:*
How to Leverage the Power of Seeing Things as They Are, 57

This is a particularly modern way of framing what mindfulness does in a culture with particular understandings and valuations of objectivity, individual autonomy, and personal choice. Now, by pointing out what I see as an underlying epistemic picture at work in modern concepts of mindfulness, I am not suggesting that practicing this way is without value, or that it is the "wrong" approach, or that it is insufficiently reflective of "traditional" Buddhist meditation. In fact, as I will elucidate later, I think there is a way in which mindfulness can enhance freedom and individual agency. For now, however, I want to point out the underlying picture and suggest some of the problems with it, thereby making space for other possibilities for framing meditation and mindfulness.

What are the problems? I need not go into all of the critiques that have been leveled against representationalist epistemologies rooted in the European Enlightenment, as well as the attendant view of the human being as a separate and distinct, autonomous individual.[7] I'll just mention a couple of issues as they relate specifically to meditative practices. Evan Thompson, coauthor of the well-known volume *The Embodied Mind* (Verela et al. 1991), characterizes the approach taken in that book as presenting mindfulness "as a special kind of inner observation of a mental stream whose phenomenal character [is] independent of such observation."[8] Much recent scientific research and scientifically inflected popular writing has been predicated on this notion, suggesting that experienced meditators might have honed their mindfulness to a point where they can, like astronomers with a particularly strong telescope, get a clearer glimpse of internal realities unknown to others. Thompson now disagrees with this way of thinking about mindfulness and argues that such efforts at inward observation inevitably alter experience and cannot serve as evidence for the nature of the experience apart from the particular kind of observation entailed in mindfulness. He cites Nyanaponika's assertion that "bare attention" leads to the discovery—a "scientific observation"—that perception appears "as a sequence of numerous and differentiated single phases following each other in quick succession"; that is, that consciousness is essentially a discontinuous process—a restatement of the Buddhist insistence on the nature of the stream of consciousness as a series of discrete moments, which is in turn essential to the nonself (*anattā*) doctrine. To which Thompson replies: "But how do we know that everyday active perception is really made up of a sequence of single phases as opposed to being a continuous flow that gets turned into a sequence of short-lived phases as a result of practicing bare attention while sitting still . . . ?" (2020, 33).[9] Rather than seeing mindfulness as a special kind of internal observation of raw, private epistemic data, Thompson now sees it as "the integrated exercise of a host of cognitive, affective, and bodily skills in situated action" (Thompson 2017, 52). This is an important step away from the model of mindfulness bound up with a notion of consciousness as a container full of private contents to be discovered through a special introspective technique, toward one that sees it as a species of embodied, enactive, social, and cultural activity. This critique reflects the broader phenomenological critique of Descartes's assumption that isolated, individual observation and logical reasoning, rather than, say, active engagement with the world or consultation with others or with tradition reveals the fundamental structures of the mind. Isolated introspective analysis is one species of inquiry that yields certain kinds of understanding, which should not be assumed to reveal the fundamental nature of mind, independent of that particular species of inquiry. The results of any inquiry are conditioned by the type of questioning (Dreyfus 1990).

This line of thinking also highlights the fact that mindfulness, rather than simply discovering a preexistent internal reality akin to the objects of physical scientific investigation—rocks, atoms, kidneys—creates novel ways of constituting oneself, the world, and the relationship between them. Cook insists that "this is a constructivist endeavor—rather than revealing a reality that is already there by 'purifying' it of the false reality effects of appearance, the work to distinguish between 'appearance' and 'reality' *creates* them as separate categories. In so doing, I suggest, a new reality is created" (Cook 2017, 115). Indeed, the very attending to consciousness in such a way as to divide it into "appearance" (judgments, emotional reactions, mind-wandering, thoughts, etc.) and "reality" (the present moment; physical sensations; the stream of thoughts itself, observed with detachment) common to some iterations of mindfulness is a specific and particular way of constituting human experience, of configuring oneself, of valuing and caring about things in a certain way, of sorting through, dividing up, nudging toward experiences that are valued, holding back from those that aren't. Such a process is deeply informed by tradition, ethical commitments, and the possibilities of thinking, feeling, and valuing offered in a particular place and time, rather than simply a non-judgmental, unbiased, neutral accessing of raw mental data. Characterizations of meditators as simply observing objective interior facts based on firsthand experience ignore the importance of the larger social context and the powerful impact on meditation practice of things like tradition, authority, faith, institutions (religious, scientific, educational, etc.), and worldview. Is it merely coincidence that meditators from Hindu traditions delve deeply into the mind and discover, after a long search, the *ātman*—the true, unchanging self—while Buddhists delve deeply into the mind and discover precisely the lack of *ātman*? I am not insisting on the strong relativist claim, here, that meditative experience will always and only mirror and amplify whatever ideas, images, and values the practitioner brings to the experience. As I will discuss later, novel experiences happen; meditators break through established categories, attain new insights, reconfigure themselves beyond established norms. Yet, the picture of the meditator as a scientist in an open-ended, value-free observation of the objective data of consciousness ignores the important role that tradition, worldview, and social context surely play in meditative practice.

The Self-as-Brain Model of Mindfulness

Scientific studies of meditation, and meditation itself, in the last few decades have been increasingly standardized and tailored to another epistemological-anthropological picture as well: what Ortega and Vidal have called the modern anthropological figure of the "cerebral subject" (Ortega and Vidal 2017) and Nikolas Rose calls the "neurochemical self" (Rose 2003), a powerful contemporary view of the human being and personhood as essentially identical with the brain and its functions. This picture depicts the fundamental nature of personhood to be constituted by the brain, such that knowledge of the self is essentially knowledge of the brain and its functions. Much of the theater-of-the-mind picture is enfolded into this one, albeit with the Cartesian ghost exorcised from the machine. The person is essentially the brain; the rest of the body is primarily a support for and instrument of the brain; the world is represented to us as stimuli entering the brain through the senses and nervous system. Our encounters with the world are bodily effects of external stimuli, represented internally. In this model, the human being is a sophisticated machine that can be tuned to greater effectiveness and worldly happiness by increased efficiency and instrumental reason. Not only has this characterization of personhood and brainhood become pervasive in popular culture and mass media—people today often say that they had a thought in their brain, instead of in their mind—it has spawned various subdisciplines and institutional practices such as neuropolitics, neuroeducation, neuromarketing, and neuroeconomics (Rose and Abi-Rached 2013).

Dispatches from the Worlds of Meditation: 2b

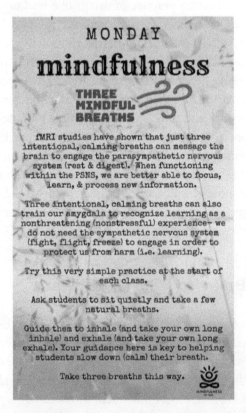

FIGURE 2.3 A "Monday Mindfulness" email sent to the Franklin & Marshall College community from the campus Mindfulness Committee. Created by Amy Faust.

This picture entails a shift from the more Cartesian-inflected model of the mindfulness practitioner as the individual self with a privileged view of subjective data of internal states—which suggests the primacy of "direct experience"—toward the idea of the primacy of the brain. On this model, what is *really* going on in the human being is flowing blood, sparking synapses, and reacting chemicals. And it is these phenomena, more than the fallible words, concepts, and the potentially illusory experience of subjects, that tell the true story. Many neuroscientific researchers on meditation still have reverence for personal experience, subjectivity, and introspection—the first-person perspective—yet hold the implicit assumption that we need confirmation by an external authority to verify that experience. The authority in this case is not the priest, the guru, or the *rōshi*, but the measuring machines—fMRI, PET scans, and EEGs.

Which brings us back to the Enlightenment Machine. Horn and Rizzuto suggest that such a machine might provide objective measures of where one is on the spectrum of experience; that it could measure, unencumbered by the ephemera of mere human judgment and guesswork, progress toward spiritually advanced states of mind; that it could trace ethical progress; that it might even be able to authenticate enlightenment itself. Such musings might sound silly to those uninterested in meditation or unfamiliar with Asian meditative, religious, and philosophical traditions. And it might well be met with eye-rolls from many neuroscientists. Nevertheless, the general idea appears to be an extension of mainstream assumptions in many neuroscientific studies that there are definitive cognitive states, the neural correlates of which are observable on imaging devices, and that these images constitute a kind of objective view into these internal states. Responsible scientists will add qualifications and hedges (popular media, less so) about just how certain and transparent this window into consciousness is, but many seem to believe that, at least in theory, machines that can pin down the exact neural correlates of mental states are possible.

The cutting edge of neuroscience itself, however, appears to be moving beyond the idea that states of consciousness, be they ordinary anger or fear or more refined meditative states, have particular "neural signatures" or "fingerprints." The "constructionist" theory of consciousness, for example, complicates the picture of mental states like emotions as having specific neural configurations occurring in specific areas of the brain, and of emotions being definitive, universal states, the same in everyone. The classical picture of emotions is that they have definite bodily and neural correlates, are universal, and are different from, or prior to, rational and conceptual processes. The constructionist theory argues that emotions are intertwined with conceptual interpretations of sensory input, which in turn are to some extent dependent on culturally available categories. One instance of fear or joy may look very different from another on brain-scanning machines, and there is no fixed neural "fear circuit" or particular region of the brain that is exclusively responsible for fear. Rather, an instance of fear is an in-the-moment construction and interpretation of what is happening based on past incidents, and a prediction of what is to come (Barrett 2017).

The idea that has been popular in neuroscientific research on meditation, therefore, that one could scan someone meditating in an fMRI machine and measure, for example, "joy" by detecting what particular region in the brain "lights up" through increased bloodflow, is becoming increasingly problematic. The notion that precise states of mind or cognitive functions, like language, fear, or mathematical calculation are precisely localized in separate areas of the brain is being displaced by the conclusion that such states and functions can come about through multiple neuronal pathways, that "most regions of the brain—even fairly small regions—appear to be activated by multiple tasks across diverse task categories" and that "the brain achieves its variety of function by using the same regions in a variety of circumstances, putting them together in different patterns of functional cooperation" (Anderson 2014, 3). The process of constructing these states of mind draws on countless possible neural configurations rather than the assigned activities of predictable, separate regions of the brain. Researchers, therefore, cannot nail down definitive neural circuitry involved even in everyday affective and cognitive states, let alone elusive meditative states described in Buddhist contemplative literature. Indeed, there is a growing critique of "neurorealism"—the credulous treating of neuroimaging as a kind of mind-reading technique that adds unwarranted credibility to an analysis or interpretation—even among neuroscientists.[10]

The constructionist theory of consciousness and the fading of the promise of precise neural correlates of mental states invites an alternative picture of meditation: rather than mindful attention apprehending uncontaminated, private contents in the mind—"anger," "fear," "joy"—states that are identical for everyone and that have definitive objective neurological patterns observable on brain-imaging technology—a more complex picture emerges. Maybe we could characterize it like this: any psychophysiological event involves a swirl of somatic signals, images, affective fluctuations, and memories that rise to meet available concepts, which solidify the experience and render it intelligible according to particular categories. These categories are not solely within the mind and thus not purely private, but are supplied by language, culture, and context. Stephen Stanley, in an article advocating a "critical-relational" perspective on mindfulness, illustrates it nicely:

> The words I am writing now are not simply my own words. While they may never have been written in precisely this order, or given this particular set of meanings, I have not invented them anew. I am using a collectively shared vocabulary which is the product of a cumulative biological, cultural and historical evolution. The meaning of the words I use arises through our complex relationships with one another over time. Specifically, through their use in a multitude of "language games" within broader "forms of life" (Wittgenstein, 1953). My words are contingent on a collective, group or interpersonal context; but this "context" is not outside of us, but rather constituted through our shared practices. (Stanley 2012, 636)

Now, I am not claiming that there is nothing to be learned through fMRI and other neurophysiological studies about how the mind or meditation work. The point significant to my own argument is that attempts through imaging and biomeasuring technology to arrive at some species of objective truth about subjective states of mind involve a certain circularity. The certainty and objectivity that seem to be conveyed by brain-imaging are, in fact, laden with ideological assumptions, culture-bound categories, and epistemic premises at the outset, as are the interpretations of such imagery. MRI machines seem to work well in diagnosing ankle fractures or adrenal tumors, but their ability to pin down the nuances of consciousness appears far more questionable. The suggestion that the machine can determine truths of the mind from outside the mind, beyond ordinary human judgment, reasoning, observation, and argument, masks the fact that the design of the machine, what it measures, and the significance of the measurements are all constructed based on—human judgment, reasoning, observation, and argument. Their authority resides in the assumptions and categories built in to the entire process of neuroimaging—assumptions and categories that are themselves culture-bound and contestable, and indeed under considerable debate today. The deference to the machine as the nonhuman (transhuman?) revealer of the neutral, unbiased truth, beyond cultural conditioning is itself conditioned by a culturally contingent epistemology. And this epistemology, wrapped up in an implicit picture of the human being as essentially the brain, engenders faith—indeed, an almost religious faith—that the machine will transcend our limitations and reveal the real; that its iconic pictures will assure us in times of doubt what we are, what we are *really* experiencing; that it will tell us whether or not we are enlightened.

Again, many, perhaps most, scientists studying meditation will be skeptical of the possibility of an Enlightenment Machine. But I'm guessing that the objections would be primarily that, first, we just don't have the technological capacity to do such a sophisticated, precise mapping of brain-states at this point, and probably won't in the near future. The second objection might be that we lack precise, replicable understandings of the things we are supposed to be able to track with such a machine, e.g., Newberg's and Waldman's "spectrum of awareness" from instinctual awareness to enlightenment or different stages of ethical or spiritual development. Both of these objections, however, still assume problematic elements of the two pictures I have presented. Both are rooted in an epistemology in which the isolated contents of the mind are observed in a private theater or represented as discrete internal states, the neural correlates of which are visualized on brain-imaging machines. These pictures, I think, are inadequate for understanding how meditation practices work in that they neglect the essential role of social and cultural context and misconstrue the ways in which individuals have introspective access to their own thoughts and feelings.

Are there alternatives to these models that might be productive? There are. Consider, for example, a philosophical understanding of consciousness rooted in the mid-twentieth-century phenomenological movement and incorporating more recent neurological and cognitive science research: the model of "embodied cognition," according to which consciousness is not solely an interior state, but a dynamic, embedded, enactive process. Alva Noë provides a nice snapshot of this perspective:

> To understand consciousness—the fact that we think and feel and that a world shows up for us—we need to look at a larger system of which the brain is only one element. Consciousness is not something the brain achieves on its own. Consciousness requires the joint operation of brain, body, and world. Indeed, consciousness is an achievement of the whole animal in its environmental context. . . . To have a mind . . . requires more than a brain. (Noë 2010, 10)

From this perspective, we can see how Thompson, also an advocate of embodied cognition, argues that mindfulness is not just the neutral observation of internal mental phenomena but also "the integrated exercise of a host of cognitive, affective, and bodily skills in situated action."[11]

In this less privatized view of cognition, the contents of the mind are not purely private; they are constructed in systemic relationship with the world— again, traditions, doctrines, ideas, common notions, affective conventions, and background concepts. The example of a well-known concept in the

Japanese language may illustrate the point. "*Mono no aware*" is a category of emotion in Japanese. It means the awareness of the beauty in fleeting things, a poignant combination of appreciation of this beauty and wistful sadness that it is so ephemeral. The fleeting cherry blossoms of spring are the quintessential illustration. Now, I am not saying that because the Japanese have a concept or term for this feeling that is absent in English, i.e., that the Japanese man in Kyoto has a possible experience available that the English woman in London does not. I just explained it in English, after all, and you likely understood it, recognized it, and remembered instances of it in your own life. Rather, because this term is a recognizable category that is developed and elaborated in Japanese art, poetry, literature, cinema, and philosophy, it is more readily available to someone immersed in that context. The swirl of indeterminacy is more likely to be drawn into the gravitational pull of a concept that has been elaborated on and refined in many cultural products that one has encountered; it is more prone to serve as a container to explain, express, nuance, and render intelligible one's experience.

This interpretation has implications for the common practice in contemporary meditation of "labeling thoughts." A popular aspect of some contemporary meditative practices is the labeling of moment-to-moment experience. Some teachers instruct students to simply notice a wondering mind, label it "thinking," and refocus attention on the breath. Others suggest a more granular approach, instructing practitioners to label phenomena with more specificity: "fear," "anxiety," "tranquility," "itching"; or perhaps even "fear of my boss," "anxiety about illness," "memory of mom." The picture I have been presenting is that mindfulness practice is not so much a matter of reflexively observing the contents of consciousness and identifying the particular thoughts or emotions as unambiguous mental states, qualia, or gestalts that are simply "there" to be discovered; rather, labeling practice entails the jumble of ambiguous sensations, images, affective fluctuations, and memories rising to meet available concepts, which solidify the experience and render it intelligible according to particular categories such that they can be labeled. The phenomenon is not merely observed but also constructed in the very process of observation. Further, there might be different possible ways of interpreting the implications of this practice. On the one hand, if the practitioner reifies the labels, seeing them as objective contents of the mind that she has discovered, she may simply be solidifying a normative conceptual framework, the dominant social imaginary of her particular cultural context, and further ensconcing herself within its taken-for-grantedness. But she might also acquire a glimpse into the process of constructing an interpretation of experience in the moment, while at the same time noticing the more indeterminate processes beneath the labels, thus getting a view into the contingency and the constructedness of such categories. This view could provide emancipatory potentials insofar as it demonstrates the fluidity and malleability of experience, thereby opening up possibilities of alternative or novel interpretations.

These ideas provide some directions for thinking through a *constructivist* understanding of meditation, which I will lay out further in the following chapters—a view of meditation not based primarily on neutral observation of internal data but on constructing particular experiences and ways of being in specific cultural worlds. Such a view sees meditation as helping practitioners construct particular ethical stances, habits of thinking and feeling, sensibilities, even political dispositions, all drawn from repertoires of possibilities available in particular cultural contexts. As we shall see, Buddhist meditation traditions also include, however, a *deconstructive* element, which keeps meditation from merely reproducing normative ways of being, thereby opening up possibilities for self-transformation in novel directions.

Meditation in Context: Initial Reflections

What difference does this more culturally inflected, constructivist view of meditation make? Here is an example. A *New York Times* opinion piece summarizing several scientific studies includes in its enumeration of the many benefits of mindfulness practice that it "shift[s] frontal brain activity toward a pattern that is associated with what cognitive scientists call positive, approach-oriented emotional states—states that make us more likely to engage the world rather than to withdraw from it" (Konnikova 2012). This conclusion that mindfulness makes us more "prosocial" is a stark contrast to the admonition in many Buddhist texts that meditators should withdraw from society, renounce family and job, and seek out isolation and solitude in a forest or cave. If you practice mindfulness in hopes of becoming more social in a culture that values sociality, you may well become more social. If you practice it in a monastic culture that emphasizes isolation and withdrawal from society, then mindfulness may well help you become *less* social. The work that meditation does, therefore, is inevitably shaped by the surrounding the ideas, aims, attitudes, and cultural context of the practitioner. Such practices do not simply produce particular, precisely reproducible mental "states" that are the same across time and space. They are part of larger ways of being in the world in particular traditions and social contexts. Researchers should keep this in mind when they make claims like mindfulness "makes" people more compassionate, more productive, or less anxious.

It may well be, of course, that similar practices have similar effects in different cultural contexts, but the surrounding interpretation of such effects
might be quite different and in ways that might have important consequences
for practitioners. For example, in classical Buddhist meditation texts, one
of the goals is the dissolution of the sense of a permanent, independent,
and substantial "self" (*attā*; Skt., *ātman*) into impersonal, component processes (*skandhas*, *dharmas*) that are not "me" or "mine." A complex system of
concepts and practices supports this goal, and meditation teachers no doubt
have long helped their students interpret such experiences as stages along the
path to awakening. In the West today, the main category available for such
experiences are pathological: depersonalization-derealization disorder.
Jared Lindahl and Willoughby Britton have documented dozens of cases
in which changes to the sense of self apparently brought on by meditation
have been distressing, impairing, or debilitating (2019). It is possible that the
lack of a rich context of interpretation, or perhaps the stark contrast of such
experiences with the normative individualistic views of the self in the modern
West, predisposes contemporary secular meditators to such experiences. As
Robert Sharf suggests:

> The depersonalization to which Buddhists aspire is not supposed to result in dys-
> functional alienation. The dissolution of the ego is meant to occur within an insti-
> tutional and ideological framework that helps one make sense of the experience.
> Nowadays, people who become depressed or depersonalized through secular-
> ized meditation practices don't have access to the conceptual resources and social
> structures to help them handle what is happening to them. (quoted in Aviv 2020)

The level of analysis that attends only to universal physiological structure
and function, therefore, cannot adequately account for how these practices
work in practitioners' lives. If we are to take seriously the first-person perspective of contemplatives, we must understand how they conceive of the
meaning, purpose, and significance of their practices in their doctrinal, social, cultural, and cosmic contexts. To understand contemplative practices
in a comprehensive way, therefore, scientific study of meditation must work
hand-in-hand with philosophers, anthropologists, sociologists, and scholars
of religion who can help articulate these contexts—and admit that there are
simply questions that cannot be addressed by the universalizing language
of the sciences. By all means we should measure what is measurable, but we
should not think that such measurements—be they oscillating brain-waves,
blood flow to various parts of the brain, respiration, etc.—get down to the
real "facts" about meditation to which all other "data" (beliefs, social situation,

cultural factors, relations of power) are extraneous. We must understand all of these factors together systemically. The study of meditation should not succumb to the modern cult of calculability in which something is only real when it is measurable and measured.

And this is why an effective Enlightenment Machine will likely never be built. It presumes at the outset the primacy of private, interior brain-states and seeks to map them with replicable precision. Yet it ignores the complex social and cultural maps that are just as important to contemplative endeavors. Such a machine promises to show us the essence of ourselves and deliver us from our human judgments, biases, misperceptions, and ideologies. Yet the machine itself represents an ideology that such disengaged neutrality is the singular road to Truth and, moreover, that such a machine could be greater than the sum of the thousands of human judgments, biases, and misperceptions that went into making it in the first place. Toward what Enlightenment would it guide seeking brains? Are there neural signatures showing a transition from refined meditative states described in traditional Buddhist texts, like consciousness of the "infinity of space" to the "infinity of thought"? The attainment of the knowledge of all past rebirths? Or would it be geared toward a Maslowian peak experience or Hindu union with Brahman? It would necessarily be programmed with its programmer's particular religious and philosophical taxonomies, which would then be encoded in the seemingly objective measure of spiritual progress and experience. Perhaps this would be a harmless neophrenological novelty, a sophisticated mood ring. Or, more worrying, a standardized measure of spiritual development prone to dogmatic control, hiding all-too-human authority and power behind the mask of the neutral, unbiased, and value-free machine.

3

What Difference Does Context Make?

Meditation and Social Imaginaries

> **Dispatches from the worlds of meditation: 3a**
> There are many wonderful communities here at the firm focusing on mindfulness and wellbeing. I started at Goldman Sachs in the Global Markets Division, and every Wednesday, a small group would meditate together in a conference room at 6:00 a.m. It was a powerful way to start the day, as that small investment of time set the intentionality and focus that would carry on well into the afternoon. We're working now with the Human Capital Management Division to put together a Mindfulness Network for the entire firm and connect those who care deeply about mindfulness and wellbeing, which I could not be more excited about.
>
> —Sarah Wood, analyst at Goldman Sachs[1]

The Work Meditation Does

Let's consider two practitioners of Buddhist meditation. The first is a contemporary Vipassana, or Insight Meditation, practitioner in the United States. She is an educated middle-class professional who earns a comfortable living and lives in a nice house with her husband and children. She attends a weekly group meditation at a Vipassana center, meditates nearly every day, and attempts to maintain mindfulness throughout her daily activities. She describes her practice as "spiritual" but also good for her physical and mental health. She is selective with her foods and occasionally practices slow, mindful eating in order to appreciate her meals, as well as her good fortune in having enough to eat. She has used mindfulness to lose weight and help her accept her body. Her view of the world is informed by science and has little room for supernatural beings, miracles, heavens, or hells. She is encouraged in her practice by studies that suggest she is building synaptic connections through her practice and changing her brain in ways that will affect her performance in

Rethinking Meditation. David L. McMahan, Oxford University Press. © Oxford University Press 2023.
DOI: 10.1093/oso/9780197661741.003.0003

many areas of her life. She tries to practice mindful communication with her family, coworkers, and friends, and it helps her to express her thoughts and feelings more clearly and less impulsively. Her practice eases the anxieties in her hectic life of negotiating a frenetic work schedule and family obligations. It helps her be more patient with her children, more compassionate with her coworkers, more focused in performing her many tasks, clearer-minded with regard to personal problems, and less likely to be overwhelmed by destructive emotions. Mindfulness helps her to focus on the present and not dwell on the past or obsess about the future. Her avocation is going to the theater and enjoying good movies and music, which she considers an integral part of her spiritual life.

Dispatches from the Worlds of Meditation: 3b

I see rich people in the world who,
because of delusion, give not the wealth they've earned.
Greedily, they hoard their riches,
yearning for ever more sensual pleasures. . . .

Sensual pleasures are diverse, sweet, delightful,
appearing in disguise they disturb the mind.
 Seeing danger in the many kinds of sensual stimulation,
I went forth, O King.

As fruit falls from a tree, so people fall,
young and old, when the body breaks up.
Seeing this, too, I went forth, O King;
the ascetic life is guaranteed to be better.

—From the *Theragāthā* 8.1, poems
by ancient Indian Buddhist monks[2]

Now let us imagine someone in the early Buddhist community for whom the wide variety of meditation and mindfulness practices were originally developed. He is a celibate, iron-age ascetic living in a forest hermitage with a few other male renunciates. He spends hours each day in various meditation exercises and has perfected many of them, though he hasn't obtained any of their extraordinary side effects, like the ability to fly or read others' thoughts. He has left behind his family, possessions, and social position in hopes of training his mind to enter a timeless, transcendent, transpersonal state beyond the endless round of birth, rebirth, and suffering—nirvana. If he cannot achieve such a lofty goal, he hopes at least to avoid rebirth as an animal, a hungry ghost, or a resident of an unbearably hot or cold hell-realm located beneath the ground. He must maintain constant vigilance against sexual impulses, laziness, restlessness, and debilitating doubts in his capacity to achieve awakening. Sexual life, having children, eating good food, enjoying physical comfort are mere temptations to be resisted. He also must maintain friendly relationships with his fellow monks, the laity he teaches and from whom he receives alms, and the powerful patrons and rulers of his area. So he has a social life, yet is constantly on guard against longing to return to the love of his parents and siblings. He eats mindfully yet is forbidden from preferring one food over another, from taking pleasure in his food, and from eating more than necessary to keep his body functioning. He is, in fact, instructed to have an attitude of disregard for all physical pleasures and to cultivate a sense of disgust for his own body. His rejection of physical pleasure extends to plays and performances, which he is forbidden to attend.

What are we to think of such radical disparities between the historical poles of Buddhist meditation? One response would be simply to dismiss modern meditation and mindfulness practices as uninformed, decontextualized, banal versions of "real" Buddhism, "original" Buddhism, or serious Buddhism. Another would be to celebrate the successful extraction of the "essence" of Buddhism by modern, rational people from the superstitious, institutional, and metaphysical traditions and from the needlessly harsh and repressive asceticism of its beginnings. A more fruitful alternative, which I wish to pursue here, is to theorize how meditation works in different cultural, religious, and historical contexts. I don't intend to make claims about the authenticity of this or that way of meditating nor to deride our modern practitioner as trivial or against the spirit of "original" Buddhism. Rather, I want to lay groundwork for understanding the work that meditation does in the lives of each practitioner; to see how context informs the meaning, significance, and purposes of these practices; to explore how the practices come to inhabit different worldviews; to examine how they foster different but overlapping skills and ways of being in the world; and to get a sense of the extraordinary and unlikely journey these practices have made between the ancient and modern worlds.

To say that cultural context matters is, for any student of sociology, anthropology, or religious studies, a rather banal statement, something these disciplines take for granted. But the most visible discourses on mindfulness and meditation practices today come from psychology, healthcare, and the sciences, especially neuroscience. There is a rapidly increasing number of academic programs at major universities, mostly in medical schools or psychology programs, that train people in mindfulness and meditation techniques. There is also a plethora of secular mindfulness and meditation programs for the general public. Mindfulness and meditation practices tracing their origins to ancient Buddhist practices have penetrated deeply into American and European culture, however vague their connections have become to the Buddhist traditions from which they have been adapted. Most representations of these practices in scientific and health-related literature, as well as in popular media, tend to interpret them as activities that float freely above culture—timeless practices that have the same significance and effects for the ancient Buddhist monk as they would for the modern professional. A great deal of the scientific research on meditation assumes that a particular meditation practice will have the same meaning, significance, and effect regardless of circumstances. Do practice A well, and it will produce mental (or brain) state X, and after continued practice, states Y and Z. If a middle-class American woman, a modern Sri Lankan lay practitioner, and an ancient Indian monk all practice it, they are all doing the same practice with the same effects and the same understanding of what they are doing and why they are doing it. This is problematic because, as I suggested in the previous chapter, meditation cannot make any sense without a rich surrounding context of ideas, social practices, cultural orientations, and ethical commitments. Such contexts inform not only practitioners' explicit understandings of what they are doing, but also their pretheoretical, tacit, implicit orientations, and even the experiences the practices generate. So, in this and the next couple chapters I want to show, first, *that* context makes a significant difference in the meaning, purpose, and effects of meditation (that's the easy part); second, *how* context makes a difference within two particular contexts (somewhat harder); and, finally, to begin to theorize meditation more generally as a technology of self or practice of self-cultivation within particular cultural, ethical, and cosmological contexts (that's the hard part).

I realize that calling Buddhist meditation a type of *self*-cultivation or technology of self will provoke, among readers who know something about Buddhism: How can we speak of these practices as constituting a kind of self-cultivation when Buddhist doctrine denies the existence of a *self*? But the way I am using this term "self" in no way contradicts the Buddhist understanding of non-self (*anātman*). Scholars are, of course, under no obligation to avoid contradicting the doctrines of the texts and traditions we explore, but in this case the notion of self-cultivation in the sense I intend happens to offer little challenge to the Buddhist insistence on the absence of a permanent, independent, partless self (*ātman*)—in fact it is broadly consistent with it. I am using the term in the sense it has been used by some modern thinkers—including other scholars of Buddhism[3]—not in the sense of assuming or trying to achieve some permanent self but more in the sense that

Michel Foucault and Pierre Hadot have used the terms "practices of self" or "technologies of self" by which "individuals are urged to constitute themselves as subjects of moral conduct" through "self-reflection, self-knowledge, self-examination, for the decipherment of the self by oneself, for the transformations that one seeks to accomplish with oneself as object" (Foucault 1978, 29). While this view of the "self" here entails self-reflection, this "is not simply 'self-awareness' but self-formation as an 'ethical subject,' a process in which the individual delimits that part of himself that will form the object of his moral practices, defines his position relative to the precept he will follow, and decides on a certain mode of being that will serve as his moral goal. And this requires him to act upon himself, to monitor, test, improve, and transform himself" (28). This "self" is a process of human subjectivity in constant flux and transformation, more a matter of activity than static being or a metaphysical essence.[4] That Buddhist practices of self-cultivation are matters of "not simply 'self-awareness' but self-formation as an 'ethical subject'" is central to my interpretation.

A further objection to thinking of Buddhist meditation as self-cultivation comes from certain very common characterizations of meditation as precisely *not* a matter of cultivating anything, doing anything, or trying to be a certain way rather than another. In this understanding, meditation is not about trying to make oneself into something that one is not but simply to observe what is present. The most important point in Buddhism, one contemporary author suggests, is "to be yourself and not try to become anything that you are not already. Buddhism is fundamentally about being in touch with your own deepest nature and letting it flow out of you unimpeded" (Kabat-Zinn 1994, 6). On this model of meditation, now quite widespread, one should forego expectations and goal-oriented behavior and simply accept what is. Some teachers, in an attempt to distinguish Buddhist meditation from New Age or psychological self-help, discourage their students from seeing meditation as a "self-improvement project."

This way of conceiving of contemplative practice does, in fact, reflect certain historical approaches to Buddhist meditation, particularly in Zen and certain Tibetan traditions, and I will address these in a later chapter. But, while the delicate balance between having goals and nonattachment to goals is a complex matter, the characterization of meditation as goalless and void of any attempt at self-improvement does not apply to the earliest historical strata of Buddhist meditation, and is also a problematic interpretation even of those traditions that seem to espouse it. In their early formation, Buddhist meditation practices had explicit goals, both distant (transcending the world entirely in the bliss of nirvana) and more proximate (fostering certain ways of being in the world). Moreover, contemporary iterations of these practices also have definite goals and cultivate particular modes of being in the world, despite various disavowals. Meditation for both ancients and moderns constitutes ways of cultivating certain ethical dispositions, sensibilities, tastes, attractions, repulsions, and indifferences. Indeed one of the primary Indic terms that gets translated "meditation" is *bhāvanā*—cultivation or creation. These practices have helped practitioners to imagine themselves and the world in particular ways, with a plethora of categories to shape one's experience and provide various techniques of self-examination and self-transformation. Far from a passive, nonconceptual, and nonjudgmental affair, many canonical descriptions of meditation require conceptual thought, judgment, imagination, and vigorous emotional engagement. They involve highly sophisticated taxonomies, ideals, and prototypes of actualized persons to contemplate and to aspire to.

If meditation practices are in many cases goal-directed, one must have concepts, models, and imaginings of what the goal is—what nirvana is, how an awakened person feels, behaves, and sees the world. Buddhist literature contains countless depictions of these, and practitioners have long been encouraged to actively contemplate them. Thus there are contemplative practices involving recollection of the Buddha's life and the lives of Buddhist saints, as well as higher worlds in which one might be reborn as a reward for living a virtuous life. There are contemplations designed to foster particular emotional dispositions, especially the four divine states (*brāhma-vihāras*): kindness, compassion, empathetic joy, and equanimity. Many meditations in the Pali literature, therefore, are future-oriented with the explicit aim of transforming the practitioner into a certain kind of person. These goals, images, and ideals form an indispensable part of the immediate context of meditation practices.

Meditation in a Social Imaginary

Despite the radical differences between the two meditators depicted above, there are commonalities: both are using techniques designed to calm the mind and foster clarity of awareness, and both either implicitly or explicitly aspire to particular ways of being in the world that include one's moment-by-moment activities as well as a broader ethical vision. Contemporary discussion and instruction on mindfulness often present it as a somewhat passive affair, a matter of "not doing," of simply observing whatever arises in the mind and letting it go, of not prescribing any particular course of action, and of clarifying the mind so that one will naturally do the compassionate and appropriate thing in whatever circumstance. Classical Buddhist texts on meditation present a more complicated picture. As we shall see in the next two chapters, contemplative practices in the Pali literature are presented as a way of constructing a particular kind of subject, a mode of self-cultivation, a way of living in the world that is intertwined with specific values, moral imperatives, ideas of the good, and notions of soteriology. Without this broader context the meditation practices are unintelligible. Yet we should not assume that contemporary secularized forms of meditation are wholly without such context—in fact, they too are surrounded by a dense web of ideas, values, and assumptions, and they too aim to create particular kinds of people with a particular ethical vision and life orientation. In the practice of our American meditator, however, much of this is in the background, an implicit rather than explicit and systematized understanding of the way things are and how a person should be. Contemporary secular and quasi-secular mindfulness and meditation practices aim to construct particular kinds of personhood that embody specific moral values, but these are in many respects quite different from those for whom these practices were designed. These meditation practices, in other words, do not speak for themselves. One can only make sense of them (either as a practitioner or a scholar) through what is external to them—the doctrinal, social, cultural, and institutional contexts into which they are incorporated.

One way of understanding this is to think about how meditation functions within a broad social imaginary. I use this term *social imaginary* to suggest a social and cultural context in which people live and make sense of their lives.[5] In the broadest sense, the social imaginary refers to the background of an intersubjectively shared lifeworld.[6] While it includes explicit intellectual ideas and moral ideals, it is, in Charles Taylor's words, "something much broader and deeper than the intellectual schemes people may entertain when they think about social reality in a disengaged mode. I am thinking, rather, of the ways people imagine their social existence, how they fit together with others, how things go on between them and their fellows, the expectations that are normally met, and the deeper normative notions and images that underlie these expectations" (Taylor 2004, 23). A few qualifications and elaborations that indicate how I am using the term:

- A social imaginary is constituted by a repertoire of concepts, attitudes, social practices, customs, ethical dispositions, institutions, power relations, and structures of authority. It includes a certain ethical vision and determines what is normative. Much of what makes up a social imaginary exists in the background rather than in explicit doctrines. It includes what is taken for granted, what goes without saying—one's default sensibilities. But I would also extend it to a cosmological context—how one imagines one's place in the world in the widest possible sense.

- It is not that everyone within a social imaginary thinks the same way; there may be a narrow or wide range in a given imaginary for individual personality types, quirks, and preferences. There will be diversity of opinion, conflict, factions, debate. But the terms of the debate are conditioned by the social imaginary.
- A social imaginary constitutes a certain horizon of what is likely to be thought, felt, and imagined, but it does not put an absolute limit on these. People rethink fundamental assumptions in light of new events and circumstances. It is not a fixed system but a repertoire of ideas and practices that are, especially today, constantly being modified, transformed, and negotiated. Any given imaginary is open-ended but not infinitely so. It encourages certain possibilities of thought, feeling, and action, and occludes others. It conditions "what comes naturally" and masks its own contingency by making its repertoire of possibilities seem like the only one, or at least the only one that makes sense. It makes what is particular to it appear universal.
- Social imaginaries are not static and might transform due to encounters with people having different social imaginaries. Practices in one imaginary enter into another and take on new significance and purposes. There may also be somewhat different social imaginaries in conflict in a particular society or communities striving to develop and articulate a novel social imaginary. (The latter, I would argue, happened in ancient India with the new ascetic movements, while the former is happening currently with regard to meditative practices.)
- A social imaginary also may extend to a particular picture of the cosmos. Especially relevant to us are the Buddhist picture of different realms of existence into which beings can be reborn—animals, gods, residents of hells, etc.—and the modern scientific cosmology, with its vast spaces, innumerable stars and galaxies, natural laws, the evolutionary development of life. Context in this widest possible sense conditions how one sees individual and social life. Different questions that impinge on personal, social, and cosmic issues are native to each of these imagined worlds, and it is obvious which kind of question belongs to which imaginary: Did I know her in a past life? Are we the only life in the galaxy? Is one's caste determined by previous actions? Can there be consciousness outside the physical structure of the brain?[7]

How does this conception of the social imaginary relate to Buddhist meditation practices? Meditation is embedded in social imaginaries and functions as a part of a larger network of practices, ideas, meanings, values, and conceptions of the good. In the broadest sense, meditation is self-cultivation within a particular social and cultural context, a particular social imaginary.

It would be far beyond the reach of this book to try and give an adequate account of early Indian Buddhist and contemporary American social imaginaries, but a brief comparison with regard to issues relevant to meditation might be useful. Let's stick with the examples I started with—the contemporary American woman and an ancient Buddhist monk. This list of terms evokes some sense of their respective social imaginaries:

Contemporary North America
individualism
freedom
self-discovery
suspicion of authority
world-affirmation
consumerism
social fragmentation
science and technology
health, happiness, stress relief, spirituality, meaningful life

Early Indian Buddhist Monastic Culture
bondage to the world
world-transcendence
karma and rebirth
renunciation of sensual pleasures, family, property, caste, sexuality
compassion, nonviolence
critique of Brahmanism and other cultural and religious traditions
urbanization

If we truly appreciate the differences between these two social imaginaries at opposite temporal ends of the history of Buddhist meditation, we will fathom something of the extraordinary journey these practices have made over the past twenty-five centuries. This brings us to the issue of change—how ideas and practices transform in their encounters with different times and places. Meditation and mindfulness practices in secular contexts—as psychological therapy, pain management, stress relief, maintenance of mental and physical health, and part of a "spiritual life" as currently conceived—are unique to our time. Contemplative practices, and any other social or religious practice, will take on new significance, meaning, and purpose depending on their cultural context. The practices themselves will change in relation to the different purposes to which they are put.

There are, of course, good reasons why some might resist this claim. First, it suggests a greater distance between the world of the Buddha and the various cultures in which Buddhist meditation is practiced today, potentially undermining claims that today's meditators are doing essentially the same thing that early Indian Buddhists (or medieval Tibetan or Tang dynasty Chan Buddhists, etc.) were doing. Second, modern authors have often asserted that meditation promises to transcend different cultures, get to the heart of the mind or reality itself, beyond contingent social arrangements, historically produced ideas, and cultural conditioning. To the first point, we should remember that these practices have been changing and developing for well over two millennia, adapting to many different places and times across Asia, picking up bits and pieces of the cultures of China, Tibet, Thailand, Japan, and others before coming to Europe and America. Although today's adaptations of Buddhist meditation are unique, it is the rule rather than the exception that such practices are constantly undergoing renovation and revision in new times and places. To the second point, I will suggest later that the very idea that meditation is about transcendence of cultural specificity and social conditioning is itself a modern and culturally specific way of thinking about it; however, it is also true that Buddhists themselves struggled with something akin to this issue, i.e., how it is that meditation gets to reality "as it is."

Further, by arguing that many contemporary people who practice Buddhist meditation are doing something *different* than their ancient predecessors, I don't mean to suggest that there is no continuity or overlap between them. It goes without saying that modern people can read Dōgen's manuals on meditation or the ancient Pali meditation texts, for example, and find much that speaks to their situation. Nor is my point that moderns are inauthentic or practicing a deficient form of meditation. There are plenty of examples of banal trivializations of Buddhist meditation practice in existence today; however, my focus is not to show how contemporary people have gotten it wrong but to try and elucidate something of how a set of practices can travel across great reaches of time and space and become transformed and renewed in novel contexts; how they can be incorporated into cultural worlds vastly different from the ones in which they were invented and be called on to address issues that could scarcely have been imagined by earlier practitioners.

PART II
MEDITATION IN CONTEXT

4
Meditation in the Pali Social Imaginary I

The Phenomenology and Ethics of Monastic Mindfulness

Dispatches from the Worlds of Meditation: 4
As if struck by a sword,
as if his head were on fire,
a monk should live the wandering life
      —mindful—
for the abandoning of sensual passion.

        **—From the *Theragāthā* 1.39, poems by ancient
        Indian Buddhist monks[1]**

I shall fasten you, mind, like an elephant at a small gate. I shall not
    incite you to evil, you net of sensual pleasure, body-born.
When fastened, you will not go, like an elephant not finding the gate
    open. Witch-mind, you will not wander again, and again, using
    force, delighting in evil.
As the strong hook-holder makes an untamed elephant, newly taken,
    turn against its will, so shall I make you turn.
As the excellent charioteer, skilled in the taming of excellent horses,
    tames a thoroughbred, so shall I, standing firm in the five powers,
    tame you.
I shall bind you with mindfulness; with purified self shall cleanse [you].
    Restrained by the yoke of energy you will not go far from here, mind.

        **—From the *Theragāthā* 5.9, poems by ancient
        Indian Buddhist monks[2]**

Rethinking Meditation. David L. McMahan, Oxford University Press. © Oxford University Press 2023.
DOI: 10.1093/oso/9780197661741.003.0004

The Historical and Cultural Context of Early Buddhist Meditative Practices

We've seen how practitioners in different social imaginaries might deploy Buddhist meditative and mindfulness practices in different ways for different purposes in order to cultivate diverse ways of being. I point out these differences not to suggest that modern meditation is a sham in comparison with some purportedly pure and authentic meditation of the past. Nor is the point to celebrate that meditation has successfully sloughed off the ancient cosmologies of the past and emerged triumphantly into the age of science, global capitalism, and the internet. I also do not want to suggest that ancient and contemporary meditators are polar opposites and share nothing in common in their respective efforts to observe and cultivate their minds. Rather, I want to understand something of the complex work these practices do in different contexts and appreciate that this work might vary in diverse cultural settings. Moreover, while the earliest meditation literature, preserved in the ancient Indic language, Pali, illustrates a striking contrast with contemporary approaches to meditative practice, it is also a source for them. That is, it constitutes one crucial stream in the genealogy of modern meditative practices. Tracing what in this ancient literature today's meditators have embraced and what they have left behind helps us understand how these practices have traveled the unlikely path from the monastery to the therapist's office.

In tracing this journey, I will be discussing some of the historical and cultural context of early Buddhism in India based on classical texts and historical studies. An important caveat, however, is that it is difficult to know what the actual practice of meditation looked like on the ground in ancient India, and the speculation in the previous chapter on what it might have been like for an ancient Buddhist monk is just that—speculation. It is important to recognize that the idealized representations we find in the normative canonical texts are not adequate guides to historical practice on the ground. My purpose, however, is not to try to get at how meditators might have *really* practiced, nor to offer a chronological history of Buddhist meditation, but instead to offer (1) a genealogy that traces certain features of meditation found in classical texts to current secularized practices that use those texts as their sources and (2) a theoretical account of how meditation is embedded in and interdependent with particular social imaginaries. Doing so allows us to notice what has been incorporated into contemporary practices from these texts and what has often been left behind or ignored. This, in turn, helps us to trace the contours of the late-modern social imaginary that has filtered out these features and, perhaps account for why this particular filtering has taken place. In this and the next chapter we dive into some aspects of Pali meditation literature, particularly the renowned *Sutta on the Foundations of Mindfulness* (*Satipaṭṭhāna Sutta*, MN 10, M i 55; henceforth, SP), to attempt to illustrate more fully the importance of the cultural context in which these practices emerged and imagine more fully the kinds of subjects these practices attempted to produce.[3]

Buddhist meditation practices arose within the broader context of various ascetic movements that constituted a broad South Asian counterculture that had become disillusioned with the dominant society and skeptical of its goals, values, and religious institutions.[4] These movements, whose adherents were called *śramaṇas*, or strivers, were austere seekers of transcendent wisdom and bliss. As many historians have pointed out, these ascetic movements arose in the context of broader changes destabilizing Indian society—pluralism, economic changes, urbanization, and the rise of larger kingdoms that gobbled up smaller ones. A monetary system was emerging along with organized trade. Often new religious movements begin in times of social change, and this is no exception. Whether in response to such changes, or to more universal human challenges, the *śramaṇas* came to take the view that life in the world could not ultimately be satisfying, and many saw it as alarmingly tenuous, plagued with uncertainty and pain. These ascetics considered marriage, progeny, sensual pleasures, labor, material accumulation, and social position to be bondage, an ensnarement in material conditions that could only bring further suffering and never lasting happiness. A passage from the Indian epic, the *Mahābhārata*, dramatizes the tension between this view and the broader, mainstream culture with a dialogue between a father and his son who wants to renounce the world and become an ascetic. The father advises:

> First, learn the Vedas, son, by living as a Vedic student. Then you should desire sons to purify your forefathers, establish the sacred fires, and offer sacrifices. Thereafter, you may enter the forest and seek to become an ascetic.

> The son retorts:
> When the world is thus afflicted and surrounded on all sides, when spears rain down, why do you pretend to speak like a wise man?

> Father:
> How is the world afflicted? And by whom is it surrounded? What are the spears that rain down? Why, you seem bent on frightening me!

> Son:
> The world is afflicted by death. It is surrounded by old age. These days and nights rain down. Why can't you understand?

When I know that death never rests, how can I wait, when I am caught in a net?

When life is shortened with each passing night, who can enjoy pleasures, when we are like fish in a shoal? . . .

Those who do good enjoy fame in this life and happiness hereafter. Foolish indeed are those who toil for the sake of son and wife, providing for the welfare by means proper and foul.

Such a man, full of desire and attached to sons and cattle, death carries away, as flood waters would a tiger sound asleep.

Death will carry away a man obsessed with amassing wealth, his desires still unfulfilled, as a tiger would a domestic beast.

"This I've done. This I must do. And that I have yet to complete." A man who is thus consumed by desires and pleasures, death will bring under its sway.

Death carries away a man who is attached to his field, shop, or house, even before he reaps the fruits of the works he has done, fruits to which he is so attached. . . .

The delight one finds in living in a village is the rope that binds. The virtuous cut it and depart, while evil-doers are unable to cut it.

Those who do not cause injury to living beings in thought, word, or deed, are themselves not oppressed by acts that harm their life or wealth. . . .

I do not injure, I seek the truth, I am free of love and hate, I remain the same in pleasure and pain, and I am safe—so I laugh at death like an immortal. (Olivelle 1995, 543–45)

The view of some of the ascetic movements was that the only solution to the world's sufferings was to stop action (*karma*) altogether. Action bound one to the world, and stopping karmic momentum would ultimately deliver one to a condition of permanent bliss beyond the body, senses, and ordinary consciousness. Desiring worldly pleasure, power, sex, status, and material goods kept one bound in a continuing cycle of birth and rebirth, in which suffering was guaranteed and satisfaction would be perpetually elusive. Accounts of the practices of Gautama Buddha's early associates involving severe mortification of the body, self-torture, and starvation reflect some of the methods thought to release the mind from the physical world. These ascetic movements also developed specific practices aimed at the complete stopping of thought and desire and the transcendence of ordinary states of mind—likely the first practices we could call "meditation."

The Buddhist teachings emerged as an alternative worldview within this already-alternative worldview of South Asian asceticism. Although the Buddhist Dharma was often referred to as the "middle way" and sought to moderate the extremes of asceticism, it was still situated within this broader ascetic worldview. This doctrine, especially in its early phases, shared the goal of the other ascetic movements, to reach an "unborn, undying" state beyond materiality and temporality, beyond what they saw as the irredeemable suffering of the world. In trying to understand the meaning and role of meditation in this social imaginary, we cannot neglect this ultimately world-rejecting dimension of the early Buddhist movement and many of its antecedents.

Yet despite their ascetic ideals and transcendent goal, the early Buddhist communities lived very much in the world. They had to eat and needed shelter; they interacted with the broader society and had communities of their own. There is no need to go into details of what is known about the social life of the early Buddhist communities except to highlight the fact that monastics were embedded in the broader society with which they shared certain general assumptions and cultural forms. The monastic community had relationships with kings, Brahmin priests, and others across the social spectrum. They had lay supporters, systems of patronage, and a variety of reciprocal relationships with the laity. Although the suttas recommend an isolated life of contemplation in the forest, many monastics spent considerable time in the cities, especially after life in monasteries became the norm. Eventually, some monasteries became wealthy and politically powerful. Monks owned property, possibly even including slaves or indentured servants, had multifaceted business arrangements, raised funds, did administrative work, and performed paid rituals for lay people (Schopen 1994, 2004). The place of meditation even in the monastic communities varied and is a matter of scholarly debate. Some evidence suggests that in ancient and medieval India, meditation was not highly valued in at least some monastic contexts, and monastics specializing in meditation were in the minority, often less esteemed than those devoted to scholarship.[5] We should not, therefore, be seduced by an idealized view, often presented in the classical texts, that the lives of Buddhist monks have been exclusively devoted to meditation and attainment of nirvana. Nor should we be tempted by the counterpart to this romanticized picture: that any Buddhist-derived practice, meditation or otherwise, that makes compromises with the political, economic, and social realities of the times is merely a degradation of the original, pure practice.

Unlike today, in ancient Indian Buddhist literature meditation was seldom recommended for addressing mundane concerns. The suttas do provide views on very worldly matters, such as how kings should rule and how a businessman should care for his money. They give advice on ordinary life in the world and advise laity on how to live more happy lives. Suttas discuss how a householder should insure a good rebirth, longevity, health, and beauty. In the *Sigālovāda Sutta*, the Buddha cautions against excessive drinking, idleness, associating with unsavory characters, and gambling. He discusses how to be a good friend, how a child should minister to his parents, how spouses should treat each other. Yet in most of the suttas' advice to the laity for what we might call living a good life—a happy life of human flourishing—one thing is conspicuously absent: meditation. Contemplative practices, it seems, were conceived in the early tradition as having primarily a transcendent soteriological goal, not the goal of helping meditators function better in the world.

There are, however, exceptions—places in the Canon where lay people are presented as meditators[6]—and there has usually been a place in Buddhist traditions for lay people who may remain married but take up monastic styles of life and therefore might meditate regularly. There are also occasional references to mindfulness practices for more "worldly" aims. Today, scholars and ardent practitioners might scoff at book titles like *Mindful Eating for Lasting Weight-Loss* (Clark 2020), but a passage in the *Doṇapāka Sutta* (S 3.13) presents the Buddha recommending precisely that. In it the Buddha observes King Pasenadi engorging himself on a meal, getting so full he is panting, and recommends mindful eating, uttering this verse to him:

> Those who always dwell in mindfulness,
> Observing measure in the food they eat,
> Find that their discomfort grows the less.
> Aging gently, life for them is long.

The king immediately hires a young man to be a kind of coach and recite the verse before every meal. Later, the king returns to show off to the Buddha his newly slimmed-down body, exclaiming: "Truly the Blessed One has doubly shown compassion for my welfare, both in this life and in the life to come!"[7] Buddhist traditions have always made space for both transcendent and mundane pursuits. While most literature on meditation is not dedicated to weight-loss or other health concerns, it does still incorporate concerns for "welfare, both in this life and in the life to come." That is, it pursues the more proximate, this-worldly goal of transforming character and improving life in this world, as well as the more distant, other-worldly goal of complete awakening and achieving nirvana.

The variety of meditation practices themselves embody this tension between welfare in this life and transcendence of the world. Some practices were oriented toward stilling the mind and abstracting awareness further and further from the senses, ordinary thoughts, concepts, and worldly phenomena in general, but many were more cognitively and emotionally engaged and pertinent to how the practitioner should live. The states of contemplative absorption (*jhānas*) are the most important examples of the former. They attempt to propel the practitioner into the "formless spheres": the spheres of infinity of space, infinity of consciousness, nothingness, and neither perception nor nonperception. Yet not all, or even most, of the great variety of meditation practices developed in early Buddhism are oriented toward such a radical abstraction from the world, and even those that were still fostered the development of particular ideas, attitudes, emotions, attractions, and repulsions.[8] *Bhāvanā*—contemplative cultivation—had to do with developing states of mind, ethical dispositions, attitudes, habits, and, yes, judgments and concepts, that were very much about how monks and nuns were to live in the world and embody the teachings of the Dharma. That such practices were ultimately aimed at exiting the world did not mean that they did not have a profound effect on structuring life within it. To the contrary, these practices were part of the construction and maintenance of an entire way of seeing the world and acting in it that was shared by its practitioners—a distinctively Buddhist social imaginary.

Meditation as Self-Cultivation in the Pali Suttas

Just Breathe

It is common to hear today that mindfulness and formal meditation should be done without goals, that it should minimize concepts and "thought," and that it is not a matter of making oneself a better person or "self-help" but simply about becoming aware of the contents of consciousness in the present moment, releasing all thought of the past and future. It may make one more ethical, but not because anyone is telling you what to do; you simply see more clearly what is good or skillful behavior and what is not and act accordingly. The Pali literature that established various Buddhist meditation practices, however, present a more complicated picture of meditation as complex, dynamic, goal-oriented, and designed to cultivate particular ideas, ethical dispositions, judgments, repulsions, and attractions—indeed to cultivate particular kinds of people. This picture might be surprising to the modern meditator for whom mindfulness of breath, staying in the moment, not judging, not doing, accepting oneself, and having no goals comprise what it means to meditate and be mindful.

The term *sati* (Skt. *smṛti*) is the Pali word most often translated as "mindfulness." In its common meaning it refers to memory or recollection. In the more technical sense it refers to close attention to a present object.[9] The most pervasive object of mindfulness in Buddhist and Buddhist-derived meditation practices today is the breath. Virtually any meditation center or monastery— not to mention therapist, doctor, or coach—teaching basic meditation will teach the aspiring practitioner to begin by relaxing the body, trying to let go of endless rumination and internal conversation, and focus the attention on the breath. Countless people throughout history in India, Tibet, China, Japan, Thailand, and more recently in Europe and the Americas, have sat down with their backs straight, focused attention on their breath, and felt the calm alertness that results. For many, this *is* meditation. Here is how the *Arittha Sutta* (S 54.6; V 314–15) introduces this technique:

> The Blessed One said: "Monks, do any of you practice mindfulness of breathing in and out?"
> Arittha replied: "I practice mindfulness of breathing in and out."
> "But how do you practice it, Arittha?"
> "Having abandoned desire for past sensual pleasures and having gotten rid of desire for future sensual pleasures, and having completely subdued perceptions of aversion regarding internal and external events, I breathe in mindfully and breathe out mindfully."

This might be the closest thing in the suttas to the standard forms of mindfulness we find today—at least it includes something like their present-moment focus. But the Buddha's response to Arittha is surprising. He continues: "There is that mindfulness of breathing in and out, Arittha. I'm not saying there isn't. But listen and pay careful attention, and I will explain how mindfulness of breathing in and out is brought in detail to its culmination." The Buddha then presents a more complicated method of mindful attention to the breath, instructing the monks to tether the breathing to various thoughts, feelings, and bodily sensations. He instructs them to sit down with crossed legs and body erect and use the breath as a vehicle to concentrate on a succession of sixteen different objects of attention. First is the breath itself, then the body as a whole, then various objects of thought and states of mind: rapture, pleasure, mental fabrication, the calming of mental fabrication, the mind, satisfying the mind, concentrating the mind, liberating the mind, impermanence, dispassion, cessation, and relinquishment. Each of these terms is like a little dharma package that opens up into a network of concepts that only make sense within the overall system of Buddhist thought. Monks would have known, for example, in contemplating impermanence, the important place that the concept has in the larger schema of the teachings, and that "relinquishment" (*paṭinissagga*) meant abandoning the destructive states of mind (*kilesa*) like greed, hatred, and ignorance.

In this text, meditators are clearly expected to have at least a basic understanding of Buddhist teachings, such that meditating on the various terms the Buddha presents opens up a cluster of ideas and categories to be contemplated during meditation. Second, the instructions certainly include attention to one's present experience, but also suggest more than just this. Arittha, who is presented as a relatively inexperienced meditator, is presumably not yet able simply to "observe" in his own direct experience of "liberation of the mind" or complete "relinquishment" of destructive states of mind—states that are essentially synonymous with awakening itself. These categories, then, are doctrines to be contemplated, ideals to be cherished, aims to be kept firmly in mind. Thus even this short sutta on following the breath presumes a dense web of doctrine, which the Buddha suggests is necessary not only as a context for practice but as an essential part of the practice itself. These are not just open-ended observations of present states of mind but also contemplations of various facets of the Dharma. The Buddha is not saying, for example, "when rapture arises, notice it," though that too might be implied. He is evoking rapture, asking the monks to consider it, to think about its place in the larger context of the Dharma—to imagine oneself in rapture, to recognize it when it happens, to be aware of it as a future possibility. In this sense he is encouraging vigorous contemplative engagement with a particular concept and recommending establishing it as a category of possible experience. All while tethering this contemplation to the movement of the breath. So it is actually a rather complicated cognitive task the Buddha is suggesting.

Rethinking the *Sutta on the Foundations of Mindfulness* (*Satipaṭṭhāna Sutta*)

It gets even more complicated in the SP, the most extensive set of instructions on meditation in the suttas.[10] A lot has been written on it, and there is no need to review it all here in order to elucidate the features I want to highlight. It will be helpful, however, to summarize the basic structure of the text. The SP lays out a series of practices and subjects that the practitioner should mindfully contemplate. It is divided into four basic parts corresponding to the four foundations of mindfulness: mindfulness of the body, feelings, mind, and objects of mind.

- A. Contemplation of the body consists of:
    1. mindfulness of breathing; contemplation of the four postures (standing, sitting, going forward, and lying down).
    2. practice of full awareness of various other bodily activities, such as moving the body in various ways, eating, and eliminating waste.
    3. attention to the foulness of the body: reviewing the physical constituents of the body, particularly the internal organs and various fluids and substances they produce.
    4. attention to the four elements within the body (earth, water, fire, and air).
    5. charnel ground contemplations: reflections on corpses in different stages of decomposition, and reminding oneself that such a fate awaits one's own body.
- B. Contemplation of feeling (*vedanā*): pleasant, unpleasant, or neutral, applied to both "worldly" and "nonworldly" feelings; then contemplation of how they arise and dissipate.
- C. Contemplation of mind (*citta*), which includes the mind in states of desire, hatred, delusion, contraction, distraction, exaltation, surpassing, concentration, and liberation, as well as the absence of all of these; then the contemplation of how these states arise and dissipate.
- D. Contemplation of objects of the mind (*dhammas*), which include:
    a. The five hindrances: sensual desire, ill-will, lethargy, restlessness and worry, and doubt.
    b. The five aggregates that constitute a human being: physical form, feelings, perception, volition, and consciousness.
    c. The six internal and external sense-bases: eyes and visual objects, ears and sounds, nose and smells, tongue and tastes, body and tangible objects, and mind and objects of thought.
    d. The seven factors of awakening – mindfulness, investigation of states, energy, joy, calm, concentration, equanimity.
    e. The four noble truths: suffering (*dukkha*), craving, cessation of suffering, and the eightfold path leading to the cessation of suffering: right understanding, intention, speech, action, livelihood, effort, mindfulness, and concentration.

The formula for observing the breath in the SP is the same as in many other suttas, using the breath as a foundation for examining other aspects of the body and bodily activities: "Breathing in long, he knows (*pajānāti*): 'I am breathing in long'; and breathing out long, he knows 'I am breathing out long'. Or breathing in short, he knows: 'I am breathing in short'; and breathing out short, he understands; 'I am breathing out short'" (M I 56). The same formula is applied to walking, standing, sitting, and lying down. Then the monk is instructed to act with "full awareness" or "clear comprehension" (*sampajañña*) when going forward, returning, looking ahead, looking away, flexing and extending the limbs, wearing robes, carrying robe and bowl, eating, drinking, tasting, defecating, urinating, walking, standing, sitting, falling asleep, waking up, talking, and keeping silent (M I 57).

What does the text mean when it recommends a kind of second-order or enhanced awareness of bodily movements—"knowing" one is walking or moving with "full awareness"? The Buddhist tradition offers a rich vocabulary for analyzing the processes of attention and awareness, presenting awareness and its enhancement through mindfulness as a layered series of phenomena. The most basic level, "orienting" (*manasikāra*)[11] denotes the simple, automatic, intentional function of the mind, the spontaneous noticing of an object or state of events. This designates our ordinary, nonreflective, half-aware functioning in the world. But the SP instructs the monk to magnify this ordinary awareness, using the term *pajānāti* (he knows, he understands). Rather than simply walking, one "knows" one is walking, focusing deliberately, intently, and explicitly on the walking to the exclusion of everything else. The key term *mindfulness* (*sati*) itself denotes a sense of deliberative attention; as Bhikkhu Bodhi puts it, a "lucid awareness" that involves "a 'bending back' of the light of consciousness upon the experiencing subject in its physical, sensory, and psychological dimensions" and "lifting them out from the twilight zone of unawareness into the light of clear cognition" (Bodhi 2011, 25). Mindfulness conveys a sense of being wide awake as opposed to absent-minded. In some texts it suggests detached observation from a distance, like the view of a person who has climbed a tower and can view a large area or cowherd watching over his cows (M I 17). In others, it is likened to a surgeon's probe or a goad that is used to tame a wild elephant (the mind) (M II 260, III 136). Finally, "full awareness" or "clear comprehension" (*sampajañña*; Skt. *saṃprajñāna*) designates discernment and the capacity to comprehend and evaluate.[12]

Bhikkhu Bodhi's analysis of these key concepts presents a somewhat different picture of mindfulness than the standard conception in contemporary circles, i.e., mindfulness as relaxed, minimally conceptual, nonjudgmental "bare attention," in which the contents of the mind are observed and accepted as they are. Instead, this knowing with lucid awareness and clear comprehension suggests not a passive observation of things but a vigorous, energetic awareness—as the sutta repeats, "ardent, alert, and mindful"—that is impossible at the level of simple, automatic awareness or "orientation." It this literature, it is not the attempt to rest in the preconceptual moment of awareness before thought and judgment kick in but an increasingly lucid apprehension of the object of awareness that opens up the possibility for considering it and judging it differently and more truly. No doubt calm and concentration are necessary for the sustained and undistracted mindful observation of phenomena, but in the SP this does not amount to passive and nonjudgmental acceptance of whatever thoughts and feelings emerge. While some meditation practices that attempt to minimize cognitive activity—especially the *jhānas*, states of concentrated absorption—the mindfulness practices in the SP and many other meditation instructions in the Pali literature often involve cognitive discernment, conceptual thought, ethical evaluation, and the explicit attempt to direct the mind in particular ways rather than others. Rather than mindfulness as "the fleeting instant of pure awareness just before you conceptualize the thing, before you identify it,"[13] Bhikkhu Bodhi points out:

There are certainly occasions when the cultivation of mindfulness requires the practitioner to suspend discrimination, evaluation, and judgment, and to adopt instead a stance of simple observation. However, to fulfill its role as an *integral* member of the eightfold path mindfulness has to work in unison with right view and right effort. This means that the practitioner of mindfulness must at times evaluate mental qualities and intended deeds, make judgments about them, and engage in purposeful action. In conjunction with right view, mindfulness enables the practitioner to distinguish wholesome qualities from unwholesome ones, good deeds from bad deeds, beneficial states of mind from harmful states. In conjunction with right effort, it promotes the removal of unwholesome mental qualities and the acquisition of wholesome qualities. (Bodhi 2011, 26–7; italics original).

Phenomenological and Psychological Reflections

To expand on our understanding of this move toward the lucid awareness recommended in the SP, it might be helpful to bring it into conversation with a few ideas in the contemporary analysis of cognition in phenomenology and cognitive science. Both of these disparate modes of inquiry are concerned with, among other things, the line between unreflective, pretheoretical activity and more explicit or complex cognition and awareness.

Philosophers in the phenomenological tradition, such as Heidegger and Merleau-Ponty, have analyzed how ordinary walking or eating, to use two of the examples from the SP, occurs in a rich context of meanings and purposes. One walks toward things, away from things, casually or formally, quickly or slowly, in places permitted or forbidden. One eats certain foods rather than others, with people of one's own group, in certain buildings or outside spaces, off certain surfaces, with a certain hand, with particular utensils. All of this, since one learned walking and eating as a child, is more or less automatic because it occurs in a context that is thoroughly internalized and requires no particular deliberation or reflection. The world presents itself to us in everyday life not as a collection of neutral things that appear first as mental representations that then acquire meaning, but as things ready-to-hand, already saturated with meanings: hammers are to be used to pound nails; a spoon is for scooping food; a doorknob beckons us to turn it and move into the next room. Things are "always already" infused with meaning, purpose, and value supplied by culture and its conventions. The world—or in phenomenological language, the *lifeworld*—is not an abstract collection of things to which we assign meanings, but a constant series of encounters, relationships, and disclosures. Things in the lifeworld draw forth our physical movements and create a momentum of physical activity that requires a plethora of implicit cultural knowledge. Once acquired, this knowledge does not appear in our everyday lives as explicit, thematic knowledge but as prereflective, tacit understanding through which we navigate our everyday existence. So in our ordinary physical activities, we can walk, eat, and use the bathroom without explicitly thematizing what we are doing. Only when we are doing something in a new way—say, learning to use chopsticks if we are accustomed to using a fork—do we need to explicitly cognize our eating. Our pretheoretical, prereflective being in the world is populated not just by ideas but by movements, gestures, and physical habits particular to that lifeworld. In this sense, moving in a different way and disrupting these movements, gestures, and habits are part of the way mindfulness practices help create a new way of being in the world. This takes effort.

Cognitive scientists and psychologists have also explored the line between automatic and effortful ways of cognizing. The "dual process theory" sees these as involving two different systems of cognition dubbed, for simplicity's sake, System 1 and System 2. Daniel Kahneman (2011) summarizes and elaborates on them in his *Thinking, Fast and Slow*:

- System 1 operates automatically and quickly, with little or no effort and no sense of voluntary control.

- System 2 allocates attention to effortful mental activities that demand it. The operations of System 2 are often associated with the subjective experience of agency, choice, and concentration. (2011, 21)

To expand a bit on this distinction: System 1 quickly creates spontaneous interpretations of events; it is the seat of associative memory and "generates impressions, feelings, and inclinations; when endorsed by System 2 these become beliefs, attitudes, and intensions" (105). It operates rapidly without much sense of conscious control or effort but also "executes skilled responses and generates skilled intuitions, after adequate training" (105). Like the phenomenologists' pretheoretical awareness, System 1 immediately recognizes a sad or angry face, effortlessly uses a fork, and generates quick impressions, intuitions, associations, feelings, and impulses.

System 2 is associated with monitoring behavior, explicit beliefs, learning something new, paying close attention, or performing complex activity. It is the seat of focused, deliberative action, ethical self-monitoring, rational judgment, and complex imaginative visualization. Although all of this would seem to suggest that System 2 is in charge—the rational agent controlling intentional activity—Kahneman argues on the basis of many psychological experiments that System 2 is also lazy and prone to depletion of energy. It takes effort to maintain its activities, and often it will simply acquiesce to the intuitive "suggestions" of System 1. When System 2 is fully engaged in a task, it is difficult to do anything else. When one is performing a complex calculation, navigating a difficult turn in dense traffic, or trying to recall a long list, it is hard to daydream or sing. The activities of System 1, in other words, are put on hold. It is also virtually impossible to do two things that require active engagement of System 2 simultaneously.

Now Kahneman admits that these the two systems are "useful fictions," "characters in a story." He is not saying there are literally two separate agents inside the mind nor two parts of the brain each in charge of these two vast divisions of labor. He is simply showing that certain activities involve "fast thinking"—intuition, impulse, quick judgments—and certain ones involve "slow thinking"—deliberation, abstract thought, control of impulses, and complicated or novel activities. How does all of this relate to meditation?

We may think that meditation and mindfulness are all about setting aside rational thought, judgment, imagination, and complex cognitive activity—just sinking into System 1 and relaxing there. Or that they are about simply being aware of whatever is happening rather than trying to "do" anything. This might well be the case in certain specific types of meditation (we'll address this in later chapters), but most of the meditations in the SP would fall definitively into Kahneman's System 2 activities. The SP instructs monastics to explicitly cognize and represent verbally the variety of physical activities that they would normally do automatically. Rather than being nonconceptually aware of the phenomenon of walking, the sutta asks the monk to explicitly verbally designate the activity, activating explicit conceptual representation—"I am walking, I am eating"—where before there was none. This enhanced awareness, at least as presented in the SP, does involve cutting off conceptual proliferation and rambling thoughts (*papañca*); nevertheless, it is not a move toward a nonconceptual state but toward more *explicit* conceptuality. Or, to put it another way, it is an opening of explicit, cognitive awareness and activity (System 2) to what is usually a flow of vague, automatic activity, carried along by deeply ingrained cultural knowledge (System 1), and apprehending it with precision, aided by conceptual and verbal characterization.

So, let's say that there is a distinction between two different systems or modes of cognition, two different nexuses of cognitive activity that have different functions. One operates without explicit attention and effort and acts more or less automatically based on skills imparted from one's surrounding culture and social norms. The other's activity requires exertion and entails more explicit, deliberative, attentive, and effortful activity. The first is prereflective and immersed in the taken-for-granted suppositions of the social imaginary, while the second *may* offer the possibility of critical reflection on these suppositions and of acting contrary to them. It seems clear that the majority of early Buddhist meditation and mindfulness practices involve the second system much more than the first. They not only entail effortful self-reflection and sustained attention, they also engage conceptual thought, evaluation, judgment, and intention.

Mindfulness and the *Habitus* of Monastic Comportment

If we consider specifically *how* these activities like walking and eating—not to mention the more complex analytical ones later in the SP—are to be reconstituted in mindfulness practice, we must attend to both the ethical and countercultural context of the early Buddhist teachings. While the distant goal of meditation and mindfulness practices was to attain awakening and transcend the cycle of rebirth, again, there are clearly more proximate goals in the SP, goals involving a radical reconfiguration of the practitioner's attitudes, ethical orientation, behavior, and overall way of seeing things—the cultivation of a very different way of being in the world than that provided by the surrounding cultural norms. Even the observation of bodily processes and activities carries an implicit ethical dimension and is part of the process of remaking the subject. The extraction of consciousness from the tacit level of habitual behavior through greater reflexivity and conceptual/linguistic designation of activities—"he *knows* that he is walking"—provides the basis for restructuring—not just deconditioning but also *reconditioning*—thought and activity along the lines of an alternative model, the Buddhist Dharma (and, more specifically, the monastic way of life). This move out of the habitual, culturally determined ways of being to a sense of self-reflexivity, a kind of meta-awareness, is crucial to the practice of mindfulness, especially in its initial development in an emerging countercultural tradition. We see in the SP an inward turn designed to disrupt and call into question the habitual ways of doing the most ordinary things—to thematize what is typically prethematic and automatic—as well as trying to reconstitute these activities with enhanced awareness.

Heidegger emphasizes how human sociality lends a kind of automaticity to action. This might help us further conceptualize the implications of such a disruption in ordinary activity in the context of early Buddhists shaping an alternative way of being. In his articulation of the "they-self" (*das man*), he analyzes how people are carried along in their ordinary lives by the all-pervasive but largely invisible force of tradition and social forms that make what we do and think automatic, habitual, and seemingly completely "natural," though they are deeply cultural. These forms are given to us invisibly so that we take certain opinions, attitudes, and ways of moving the body as simply what "they"—meaning all of us—do without reflection. According to Heidegger, people live most of their lives immersed in this prereflective anonymity of the they-self and its tranquilizing sense of inevitability.

> We take pleasure and enjoy ourselves as *they* take pleasure; we read, see, and judge about literature and art as *they* see and judge; likewise we shrink back from the "great mass" as *they* shrink back; we find "shocking" what *they* find shocking. The "they," which is nothing definite, and which all are, though not as the sum, prescribes the kind of Being of everydayness. (1962 [1927], 164)

For Heidegger what awakens a person from the habitual familiarity of the they-self is a crisis of anxiety in which its familiar patterned activity and thought are disrupted, thus laying bare the contingency of what was once taken for granted.[14] On this model, part of what the mindfulness and meditation practices of the SP were doing was to disrupt the familiar sense of even the simplest activities as part of a larger process of extracting the monastics from their identities as laypeople, identities taken for granted as a part of the particular "they-self," and to reconfigure these identities as monastic followers of the Buddha's Dharma with different sensibilities, comportment, and ideas.

Part of the rationale for the observation of the body has an important function in developing analytical knowledge of the microprocesses of human experience. It was believed to reveal the hidden, underlying component processes of activities as a part of the broader project of coming to understand the human being as a causally constituted network of events rather than a static, independent entity. There is also an ethical component to it that I want to develop further, and it is tied to attitudes and behaviors regarding the senses and sensual experience. In modern articulations of mindfulness, one reason to be mindful of one's activities might be to gain a greater appreciation of them and of one's life in general. We enjoy our lives more when we notice the subtle textures and flavors of our food, the nuances of the sensations of our body when we walk. Mindfulness allows us to slow down and appreciate the beauty and wonder of the world. But here, the reader of modern Dharma books will find something unexpected. If *appreciation* (a subject that we will expand on in chapter 8) is a key term in modern meditation movements, something different is going on in the ancient Indian tradition. Monastics were specifically instructed *not* to relish their food, physical beauty, or any other sensual pleasure. With regard to all pleasures of the senses, even the most subtle, the aim was in fact to become "disenchanted" (*nibbidā*) by them and always on guard against being taken in by them:

> On seeing form with the eye, [the monk] does not grasp at its signs and features. Since, if he left the eye faculty unguarded, evil unwholesome states of longing and dejection might invade him, he practices the way of restraint, he guards the eye faculty, he undertakes the restraint of the eye faculty. . . . On smelling an odor with the nose . . . . On hearing a sound with his ear . . . . On tasting a flavor with the tongue . . . . On feeling a tactile object with the body . . . . On cognizing a mental phenomenon with the mind, he does not grasp at its signs and features. (Bodhi 1995, 246 [M 27; I 175–84])
>
> What accords with the Dhamma is this: that he keep cultivating disenchantment with regard to form, that he keep cultivating disenchantment with regard to feeling, that he keep cultivating disenchantment with regard to perception, that he keep cultivating disenchantment with regard to fabrications, that he keep cultivating disenchantment with regard to consciousness.[15]

If we are to keep to the historical context of the early Buddhists and understand the challenges of monastic living, we must conclude that part of the purpose of becoming aware of the body and its movements, impulses, and activities was to discipline and gain more control over the temptation to be "enchanted" by sense objects. This continued vigilance (*appamāda*) and discipline were necessary, in part, simply because doing the things required of a monastic—abstaining from all sexual activity, resisting sensual pleasures like eating after noon or indulging in physical comforts—were difficult. But it also involved a complex process of reconfiguring and transforming a person thoroughly, both as an individual and as a member of a highly specialized community. The ordinary movements of the body and habits of mind needed to get along—walking and eating—always come laden with context-dependent meanings. To do something radically different required a disruption of the tacit level of experience (System 1 in Kahneman's terminology) in order to bring every activity to explicit cognition and intentional direction (System 2). Only then was it possible to gain more control over and transform this deep, habitual way of being in the world, not to mention the biological urges to sex, indulgence in food, and other luxuries forbidden the monk. If one is to vigilantly observe all of one's movements, explicitly cognizing and labeling them, one is less likely to let one's hands drift toward a forbidden evening meal or prohibited sexual activities. Constant attention to the body, mind, feelings, and objects, therefore, not only was directed toward cognizing their true nature, it was also part of being on guard against the impulse to break monastic ethical commitments. We can deduce this from the many rules laid out for monks and nuns in the Vinaya literature and the repeated emphasis in the suttas on being constantly heedful, vigilant, and disciplined. Bodies were a particular locus of this discipline.

So if mindfulness of the breath harnesses attention, mindfulness of the basic movements of the body, "knowing one is walking," etc., is not only an explicit awareness of what was once hidden by its utter familiarity—the habitual flow of experience and activity—it also constitutes the possibility of reconfiguring this activity, of reinterpreting its significance, of giving it a new meaning and performing it differently. It suggests not just attention to walking itself but also how one *should* walk how one *should* eat according to the many regulations a monastic takes on. A brief look at just some of these regulations from the *Pāṭimokkha* makes clear why mindfulness was a necessary part of every meal for the monastic:

32. I will eat almsfood methodically .... 35. I will not eat almsfood taking mouthfuls from a heap .... 36. I will not hide bean curry and foods with rice out of a desire to get more .... 37. I will not look at another's bowl intent on finding fault .... 39. I will not take an extra-large mouthful .... 40. I will make a rounded mouthful .... 41.

I will not open the mouth when the mouthful has yet to be brought to it . . . . 42. I will not insert the whole hand into the mouth while eating . . . . 43. I will not speak with the mouth full of food . . . . 44. I will not eat from lifted balls of food . . . . 45. I will not eat nibbling at mouthfuls of food . . . . 46. I will not eat stuffing out the cheeks . . . . 47. I will not eat shaking (food off) the hand . . . . 48. I will not eat scattering lumps of rice about . . . . 49. I will not eat sticking out the tongue . . . . 50. I will not eat smacking the lips . . . . 51. I will not eat making a slurping noise . . . . 52. I will not eat licking the hands . . . . 53. I will not eat licking the bowl . . . . 54. I will not eat licking the lips . . . . 55. I will not accept a water vessel with a hand soiled by food . . . . 56. I will not, in an inhabited area, throw away bowl-rinsing water that has grains of rice in it.[16]

Other forbidden bodily practices include, for example, walking with arms swinging or flailing, or walking tiptoe or on one's heels—and, of course, an extensive inventory of sexual acts. Although mindfulness for monastics entailed self-reflexive observation of whatever they happened to be doing, it was also an essential ingredient in radically changing what they were doing and how they were doing it. It meant cultivating the attention necessary to take rigorous control over the most minute actions. It involved acquiring a certain way of bodily being, a certain etiquette proper to a monastic. Cultivating mindfulness, therefore, was intertwined with cultivating virtue.

Now, I am not suggesting that mindfulness in this context is merely about obeying trivial rules. Rather, I am suggesting that trivial rules are not trivial in this case but, rather, are important ways of embodying what the tradition considers an awakened person's way of being in the world. Comporting oneself in this manner makes it more likely that one will *become* such a person. And it is not only rules of restraint that are important in this process. The monastic is to cultivate many ethical virtues: kindness, compassion, patience, fairness, honesty. Monks are instructed to look upon one another "with kind eyes" and regard all beings as a loving mother sees her child. Monastic training, therefore, creates an entire culture, an ensemble of physical, emotional, ethical, and intellectual dispositions.

One way to think about what is going on here is that monastics are creating a particular *habitus*, that is, a system of durable dispositions and habits through which one responds to the world spontaneously (Bourdieu 1977). In Saba Mahmood's reworking of the concept, *habitus* refers to a "specific pedagogical process by which moral virtues are acquired through a coordination of outward behavior (e.g. bodily acts, social demeanor) with inward dispositions (e.g., emotional states, thoughts, intentions)." *Habitus* in this usage refers to "a conscious effort at reorienting desires, brought about by the concordance of inward motives, outward actions, inclinations, and emotional states through the repeated practice of virtuous deeds" (2001, 215). In this sense, Mahmood suggests, "action does not issue forth from natural feelings but *creates* them. Furthermore, it is through repeated bodily acts that one trains one's memory, desire, and intellect to behave according to established standards of conduct" (214).

In the common modern understanding of agency, the autonomous individual determines consciously to do something, and the outward behavior is an expression of that inward intention. To do something other than that is insincere or deceptive. Ancient technologies of self (and some contemporary ones as well), however, often emphasize the repeated, disciplined *performance* of the details of virtue as a way of training the inward dispositions to follow the performance. The physical dimensions of monastic mindfulness in the Pali social imaginary—bringing attention the ordinary details of walking, moving, eating, etc.—provide an initial break with the habitual order of bodily comportment in order to provide alternative ways of walking, moving, and eating—that is, the way of a buddha. This opens the door to the more complex revaluing and transforming of the emotions, thoughts, ethical comportment, and states of mind.

These reflections help us begin to theorize a different way of considering the relationship between meditative practices and culture than that which has taken hold today. Rather than taking for granted the sovereign, interior self that represents, assesses, reacts to, or detaches from an external world, it suggests subjectivity as an interwoven, enactive, embodied process in systemic relationship with external objects and cultural forces. In the next chapter, we further examine some of the corporeal and cognitive dimensions of mindfulness in the Pali imaginary and further develop this interpretation.

5

Meditation in the Pali Social Imaginary II

Corporeal and Cognitive Mindfulness

Dispatches from the Worlds of Meditation: 5
Police Mortuary. St. Francis St. (Off Kinsey Rd.) It is situated in the small
St Francis Street behind the Medical College (which is opposite the SE
corner of the General Hospital complex.) This police morgue is suitable for practicing the *asubha-kammaṭṭhāna* [contemplation of the
impure]. Bhikkhus normally do not need to get official permission to
enter here and they can walk in and have a look. (Otherwise, ask permission from the director, Dr. Alwis, or from one of the anatomists.
The monk at the nearby Central Hospital Vajirāmāya—see above—
can help too.) There is very poor hygiene and one needs to be careful.
Don't go bare-footed into the cutting theaters as there are scalpels,
blood stains, etc., on the floor. Afterwards one will need to wash all
one's robes to get rid of the odour. Open on all days, but on Saturday
and Sundays only in the morning. Old corpses in various stages of
decay are in the cool-cells next to the main autopsy room and can be
viewed too. Nearby, off Kinsey Road on the backside of the Hospital, is
the Hospital Mortuary where autopsies are also done.

**—From "Information about Meditation Centers, Forest
Monasteries, and other important places in Sri Lanka for
Western bhikkhus and serious lay practitioners," compiled by a
Theravāda Buddhist forest monk living near Kandy[1]**

The Body: As It Is

We have examined some aspects of the role of mindfulness in bodily comportment in the SP and other early Buddhist meditative texts. But these texts
also deal with restructuring cognition and affect, and these instructions also
begin by addressing the body, i.e., how to see it and feel about it. Bodies have

Rethinking Meditation. David L. McMahan, Oxford University Press. © Oxford University Press 2023.
DOI: 10.1093/oso/9780197661741.003.0005

long been a locus of attention in Buddhist and Buddhist-derived meditative practices. The significance given to bodies, however, diverges considerably in ancient Buddhist contexts and mindfulness in the contemporary world-affirming, body-affirming culture of Europe and North America.

The "body scan" has become a very popular technique in contemporary mindfulness meditation. It is taught in mindfulness retreats, therapy sessions, and classes in hospitals, universities, and health clubs. In his influential account, Jon Kabat-Zinn frames the practice in the context of American society's obsessive concern with body image, which he says often leads to a "deep-seated insecurity about our bodies" and the feeling that they are "too fat or too short or too tall or too old or too 'ugly'" (2013 [1990] 75–6). The body scan, he says, is about "*experiencing* our body" in contrast to an "overlay of judgmental *thinking about* the body" (76, italics original). In order to appreciate the body—"how wonderful it is to have a body in the first place"—one must "tune in to your body and be mindful of it without judging it" (76). The body scan involves lying on one's back and focusing attention, coordinated with the breath, on each successive part of the body beginning with the feet and slowly, calmly working the attention up to the head. Kabat-Zinn's instructions take forty-five minutes to complete. Some instructions say to release tension in the various parts of the body to which one is attending. By the end, one is to feel a deep sense of relaxation and well-being, with minimal conceptual and discursive thought. Therapists and mindfulness teachers routinely teach this technique as a way of addressing insomnia, stress, anxiety, body-image problems, pain management, and a host of other psychological and physiological problems. Researchers have amassed a great deal of evidence for its effectiveness, and it has undoubtedly brought benefit to many.

Many contemporary mindfulness teachers today are likely unaware that the source of this practice is the third set of contemplations of the body in the *Sutta on the Foundations of Mindfulness* (SP). A glance at the original body scan reveals that its content, significance, and meaning could hardly be more different from its contemporary iteration. It begins, much like the contemporary practice, with the instruction to "scan the body from head to feet." But rather than simply instructing the practitioner to scan over ankles, knees, arms, etc., it dwells on the internal, asking the meditator to imagine his or her internal organs and bodily fluids, noting that they are "full of impurity":

In this body there are head-hairs, body-hairs, nails, teeth, skin, flesh, sinews, bones, bone-marrow, kidneys, heart, liver, diaphragm, spleen, lungs, large intestines, small intestines, contents of the stomach, faces, bile, phlegm, pus, blood, sweat, fat, tears, grease, spittle, snot, oil of the joints, and urine. (Bodhi 1995, 147 [M I 57])

Clearly the intent here is not to provide a relaxing, noncognitive exercise in calming the mind and body but to inculcate a particular way of seeing the body. The manner of viewing the body suggested in this contemplation, it should be noted, does not overturn the dominant ways of understanding things in the Brahmanical context, as do some Buddhist meditation practices, but rather exaggerates them. Ancient India was a society quite concerned with purity and pollution, and among the most polluting things were bodily fluids and internal substances. Pollution by such substances was of particular concern to members of high castes, who could be polluted not only by bodily substances but by even casual contact with those of lower castes. It is likely that all human beings have a natural aversion, bequeathed by evolution, to potentially pathogenic blood, pus, urine, and the like. But these have carried a particular significance in Indian culture, as evidenced by the elaborate prohibitions on contact with them and rituals of purification required after contact. The corporeal contemplation in the SP is thus designed to foster revulsion through imagining what many meditators had probably never seen—the insides of the human body. This visualization is also a cognition of something obviously true—that the body does, in fact, contain viscera, blood, bile, and so on. But this is also an act of imagination that reveals another perspective usually concealed literally beneath the skin, yet also figuratively behind the tacit notion that bodily purity is secured by washing, whether by ritual bathing or simple cleansing. This purity, the text implies, is an illusion, for no matter how clean one's skin, inside is concealed all manner of foulness beyond reach of purification.

This contemplation moves beyond the first two—attention to the breath and physical movements—in several ways. It is not just a method of bringing greater awareness to bodily sensations, activities, and processes. It is a move toward the crucial concept of insight (*vipassanā*). Here we have to examine this concept more thoroughly, and in a way that goes against the grain of some modern interpretations. The picture often presented in modern meditation literature is that bare attention to the object of contemplation leads to elimination of concepts to reveal the thing "as it is" (*yathā-bhūta*), shorn of all cultural conditioning, biases, and emotional entanglements. Some authors have interpreted this as insight into the unconditioned, ultimate truth, beyond language, concepts, and doctrine. Yet insight in this case is highly contextual, saturated with values, judgments, doctrine, and ethical implications. Rather than a neutral description of the body to calmly and nonevaluatively contemplate, our text presents a highly charged imaginative exercise bringing forth image after image specifically intended to create a visceral sense of revulsion. If this intent is not clear from the SP itself, it should be from the earlier *Vijāya Sutta*

(S 1.11), on which this part of the SP is likely based. Telling the reader that the body is typically not seen "as it is" (*yathā-bhūta*) the narrator goes through all aspects of the body that the SP mentions—blood, phlegm, pus, etc.—then insists: "The fool, beset by ignorance, thinks it beautiful." The monk who has seen the body "as it is," therefore, "should let desire for the body fade away":

> This two-footed, filthy, evil-smelling,
> filled-with-various-carcasses,
> oozing-out-here-&-there body:
> Whoever would think,
> on the basis of a body like this,
> to exalt himself or disparage another:
> What is that
> if not blindness?[2]

   Clearly insight in this case is not a matter of bare, nonconceptual attention, much less value-free objectivity. The insight into the body that these passages attempt to foster undercuts another, more typical, way of seeing it: as beautiful, worthy of producing vanity or lust. This more typical seeing is, according to the sutta, "blindness." True seeing requires seeing into the body, an imaginative recreation of what we know lurks inside, revealing another aspect not usually considered. Far from attempting to alleviate our "deep-seated insecurity about our bodies," as Kabat-Zinn puts it, this contemplation seems intent on exacerbating it. The point is to characterize the body in a particular way, to highlight one aspect rather than another in order to suggest a superior way of understanding conducive to following the Dharma. Seeing the body "as it is" in this sense is less an ontological statement of things in their ultimate nature than a statement suggesting an attitudinal and ethical stance—an alternative imagining of the body and its significance. It does not assert that there are no beautiful bodies but, rather, highlights their occluded aspects—aspects far more important for practicing the Buddhist path, especially for celibate monks. Nor is "knowing" the body in this sense used to indicate knowing a general, metaphysical truth but, instead, an interpretation of specific phenomena in accordance with the Buddha's teachings. The insight here has to do not with discovering a stable bedrock of truth beneath delusional conceptions but with providing a perspective more conducive to the monastics' moral commitments and soteriological goal. This way of *valuing* (or rather, devaluing) the body and its implications was meant to apply to everyone—everyone has insides and will die—but it is especially relevant to monastics, whose vows put stricter limits on their bodily activities.

Corporeal Crisis

Dispatches from the Worlds of Meditation: 5b
This swarthy woman
[preparing a corpse for cremation]
        —crow-like, enormous—
breaking a thigh & then the other thigh,
breaking an arm & then the other arm,
cracking open the head, like a pot of curds,
she sits with them heaped up beside her.

Whoever, unknowing, makes acquisitions
        —the fool—
returns over & over to suffering & stress.
So, discerning, don't make acquisitions.
May I never lie with my head cracked open again.
                                    —*Theragāthā* 2.16[3]

Although it is, again, difficult to know how monks practiced in ancient India, something like the following likely happened many times. A monk walks slowly out of the monastery. He is nervous, embarking on this endeavor for the first time. The closer he gets to his destination, the more trepidation he feels. He notices a tightening in his stomach and uses mindfulness techniques he has been taught to calm his nerves. He smells his destination before he sees it; wood-smoke combined with a hint of putrefying flesh. He begins to hear the chanting of the priest performing funeral rights, the crackle of flames, the gentle lapping of the river on the banks. The first peaks of flame appear from a roaring pyre, while others are smoldering mounds of ash. A man with a basket filled with ash slowly wades into the river and sets the contents loose in the water, adding to the immense black stain spreading across its surface. The monk finds a body likely left by a family with no means to pay for cremation. Slowly he takes his seat in front of it, crossing his legs, straightening his back, and fixing his gaze firmly on the corpse. The practice is not confined to the ancient world, as Dispatches 5a, at the beginning of this chapter, shows.

The contemplation of corpses is the final stage of mindfulness of the body in the SP, the "cremation ground contemplations." If the earlier contemplations were meant to disrupt habitual and pleasant ways of seeing the body, this one provides a more jarring disruption. The monk is instructed to go to the charnel ground, where the dead are brought for cremation, or to imagine such a scene.

Again, bhikkhus, as though he were to see a corpse thrown aside in a charnel ground, one, two, or three days dead, bloated, livid, and oozing matter, a bhikkhu compares this same body with it thus: "This body too is of the same nature, it will be like that, it is not exempt from that fate." (Bodhi 1995, 149 [M I 58])

The monks are then instructed to observe or imagine bodies in various stages of decomposition: devoured by birds, wild animals, and worms; reduced to a skeleton containing diminishing amounts of flesh; bones scattered here and there; and, finally, bones crumbled to dust. In each case, the monks are to remind themselves that their own bodies too will suffer such a fate (Figure 5.1).

It might be surprising that people of ancient India should have to be reminded of their mortality. Surely premature death would have been more frequent and familiar than in contemporary societies. Nevertheless, many authors from the ancient world have attested to a certain blindness to the realities of death—at least one's own. In the legends of the Buddha, the crisis that precipitates the young Gautama's becoming disillusioned with palace life and leaving home for the life of an ascetic is his first encounter with old age, sickness, and death—the latter in the form of a corpse being carried to the cremation ground.

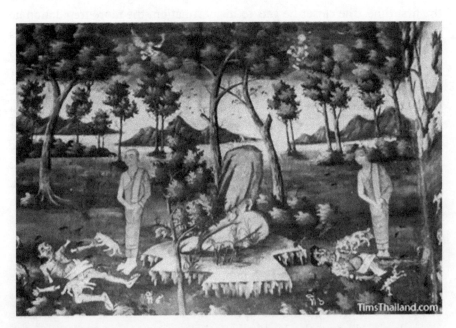

FIGURE 5.1 Painting of corpse contemplation at Wat Um Long in Thoen, Lampang province, Thailand. Photo by Tim Bewer.

This practice cultivates the explicit consciousness of the inevitability of death as an intervention in the unreflective life that takes for granted life's indefinite continuation. It attempts to dispel a psychological illusion in order to realize—to make real for oneself by vivid imagination and explicit conceptualization—a truth that everyone knows but, the text implies, few fully comprehend. As with the previous contemplations of the body, these are designed not only to disrupt a habitual way of understanding things but to supply an alternative vision, along with an implicit demand for action. It combines vivid, shocking imagery with cool anatomical realism to create a sense of urgency that would echo throughout Buddhist literature and practice in Asia. The encounter with death as a way of motivating determination to pursue liberation is a leitmotif in far-flung Buddhist traditions. Tibetan texts routinely remind readers of the "precious human life," the inevitability of death, and the uncertainty of its time. A liturgical verse recited in in Zen monasteries reiterates the same point: "Let me respectfully remind you, Life and death are of supreme importance. / Time passes by swiftly and opportunity is lost. / Each of us should strive to awaken. / Awaken! Take heed! Do not squander your life." Far from a serene contemplation promoting acceptance of one's mortality, such reflections on death are, as Donald Lopez suggests, more a matter of stress *induction* than stress reduction (2012, 108)! Such vivid evocations of the extraordinary fragility of human life appear designed to provoke a crisis of anxiety that spurs one to practice the Dharma with one's entire being.

The modern interpretation of the cremation ground meditations has been that this heightening of the awareness of mortality is ultimately life-affirming, increasing one's appreciation of the precious and fleeting human life. Of course we cannot know all of the effects that these contemplations had on monastics in ancient India—they may well have experienced a sense of this appreciation that modern people have, watching the smoke rise from cremation pyres or gazing at birds picking at corpses. The texts, however, don't speak of appreciation but, again, of disenchantment. Appreciating the "precious human life," as a standard Tibetan formula goes, is a matter of contemplating, first, the rarity of human birth, which was considered to be uniquely advantageous to achieving awakening. Unlike an animal, a human is intelligent enough to understand and follow the Dharma. And unlike the gods, humans have enough suffering that they are motivated to follow it. Buddhist teaching considers the human rebirth rare, and life during the time when a Buddha's Dharma still survives even rarer. Those who squander this opportunity risk eons of roaming in *saṃsāra* before being born as a human again. This is quite different from the modern life-affirming ethos, which takes embodied human life as a good in and of itself, to be cherished, celebrated, and nurtured for its own sake. Yet this does not mean that Buddhism entails gloomy, world-negating pessimism: the Buddhist position on the possibility of overcoming all suffering by attaining the eternal bliss of nirvana is in fact wildly optimistic. But we should also not confuse it with modern attitudes about the cherishing every moment one is granted so that one can treasure family, food, and a good novel. The suttas do not suggest cherishing one's life but renouncing it for a higher sense of life. Nor were they suggesting by highlighting the decay of the body that one should accept with equanimity the relentless forward momentum of time, ageing, and death. Rather, the suttas suggest that these were unacceptable and must be overcome through great effort.

Dispatches from the Worlds of meditation: 5c

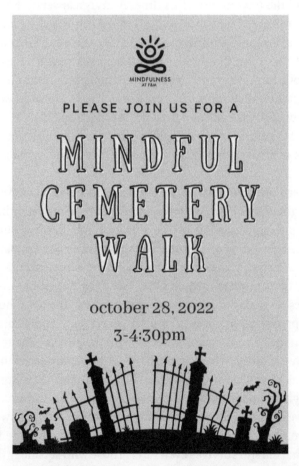

FIGURE 5.2 An email sent to the Franklin & Marshall College community from the campus Mindfulness Committee. Created by Louise LoBello.

Doctrinal Contemplations

The remaining meditations in the SP are more explicitly cognitive, doc-trinal, and analytical. They intertwine taxonomies of mind and its objects with injunctions on how one should behave, what states of mind should be fostered, which struggled against. Now the text instructs the practitioner to observe feelings (*vedanā*), which are categorized as pleasant, unpleasant, or neither. The semantic range of this term is different than the English "feeling" or "emotion" (Heim 2021). It refers to a basic attraction or repulsion, a good, bad, or neutral feeling upon encountering anything whatsoever, a person, place, thought, memory, etc. Again, one is to "know" one is feeling these things—"I am experiencing a pleasant feeling," "I am experiencing an un-pleasant feeling"—and note their arising and passing away. Finally, one notes, simply, "this is a feeling" and dwells "unattached." Similarly, the text instructs the practitioner to contemplate the mind (*citta*) in states of desire, hatred, de-lusion, contraction, distraction, exaltation, surpassing, concentration, and liberation, as well as the absence of all of these, observing their arising and dissipation.

The sutta then directs the monk to observe (*anupassati*) the various feelings and mind-states, noticing the fact that they arise and disappear, thus drawing attention to their transience. It also provides a taxonomy of feelings and states of mind, thereby erecting a framework for directing and shaping thought and affect in particular ways. This exercise is not a free-form observation of what-ever states of mind emerge but an evocation of particular ones to be observed and analyzed. Nor is this simply a neutral taxonomy; instead, the states are valued in particular ways: desire, hatred, delusion, and distraction are obvi-ously to be avoided, while exaltation, surpassing, concentration, and liberation are to be fostered. Likewise, the text directs the practitioner to contemplate the five hindrances—sensual desire, ill-will, lethargy, restlessness and worry, and doubt—and to actualize the seven factors of awakening: mindfulness, in-vestigation of states, energy, joy, calm, concentration, and equanimity.

If these contemplations deal primarily with states of mind to be fostered or overcome, the next contemplations—of the senses, sense objects, and the five aggregates—have more to do with creating a picture of what the human being—and the world itself—*is*. Yet this is also intertwined inevitably with what one should *do*. These contemplations are distinctively analytical in the sense that they take supposed wholes and break them down into parts. This is a crucial element of the early Buddhist picture of reality. Everything is made up of transient processes conditioned from the past, and nothing permanent or stable is to be found in this world. Yet the human capacity for establishing fixed concepts produces the illusion that we live among static, independent realities. Words seem to refer to independent things in the world, and once things are taken as fixed and stable, they become the basis for clinging, aversion, and frustration. According to Pali Buddhism, the things that words name are not independent realities but collections of the fundamental constituents of experience, called *dharmas* (Pali: *dhammas*).[4] These are momentary events, whose patterns create the appearance of stable entities when they are conceptualized. Yet the entities that we take to be independent things or beings are actually fluid, composite, plural, and causally conditioned processes that are constantly moving, forming, breaking up. Meditative insight allows the practitioner to break through the reification imposed on this process and see things as they truly are—an interdependent, constantly moving succession with no stable entities and nothing to hang on to.

Perhaps the most consequential of these illusory wholes is the self (Pali: *attā*; Skt: *ātman*). Some of the ascetic traditions contemporary with early Buddhism strove to find a permanent, transcendent self beyond change and suffering. Early Buddhists found this quest misguided, believing that attributing "self"—in the sense of permanence, immutability, independence—to anything in the world was a mistake. Instead, they analyzed what was normally considered to be self into constituent component processes. The idea, in its most general sense, is that we mistakenly attribute a sense of unity and permanence to things that are composite and impermanent. We then become attracted, repelled, or otherwise emotionally entangled in these shadowy realities, creating suffering and bondage. Seeing through these artificial unities, be they one's "self" or various objects in the world, allows the practitioner to apprehend the underlying plurality and transience of things. Meditative insight, therefore, is often characterized as seeing in all things impermanence, lack of self, and inability to bring about satisfaction. Contemplation of the five aggregates (Pali: *khandas*; Skt: *skandhas*)—the five processes we mistake for a permanent self: physical form, feelings, perceptions, volition, and consciousness—is perhaps the quintessential example of cultivating penetrating insight because it addresses one's very person. In this contemplation one is asked to re-envision oneself not as a stable, enduring, unitary, independent being, but as a fluctuating, intertwined combination of various processes continually arising and passing away. Likewise, the apparent unity of experience is broken down in an alternative way with the analysis of the sense capacities (seeing, hearing, tasting, smelling, touching, and thinking) and sense objects. Meditation on nonself invites the practitioner to reimagine oneself as plural and processual rather than unitary and stable.

The final contemplation in the SP is on the well-known summary of the Dharma purported to be the contents of the Buddha's first public talk: the four truths of the noble ones, more commonly known as the Four Noble Truths, and the Eightfold Path. It gives an analysis of the basic problem human beings face—suffering caused by craving for things that cannot satisfy—pronounces the possibility of the overcoming of suffering and craving (*nibbāna*; Skt.: *nirvāṇa*), and elucidates the path to this liberation: right understanding, intention, speech, action, livelihood, effort, mindfulness, and concentration. This contemplation is not a matter of fine-tuned observation of the movements of consciousness, nor a breaking down of conceptual wholes into their *dhammas* (Skt. *dharmas*), but rather a conceptual reflection on the essentials of the Dharma—the immersion in a set of ethical injunctions, attitudes, ideas, and practices that, despite its remote and otherworldly goal, constitute a comprehensive way of being in the world. It includes learning, judgments of right and wrong, cultivation of particular attitudes and dispositions, planning for the future, and remembering the past (especially the Buddha and his teachings).

Rethinking the Foundations of Mindfulness

By the end of the sutta the reader has encountered a sketch of the fundamentals of Buddhist doctrine and practice; a basic picture of what a human being is in its components and functions; suggestions on attitudes to take toward various things, for example, the body (it is repulsive rather than attractive, it will decay rather than endure); lists of what mental and emotional states to become familiar with, as well as which to avoid and which to embrace; a diagnosis of the essential problem of human life (suffering and craving); and the comprehensive set of attitudes, ethical injunctions, and practices that guide how a follower of the Dharma should think and behave (the Eightfold Path). The SP, therefore, is at once a summary of how a follower of the Buddhist Dharma should learn to see the world and a set of practices to habituate the mind to seeing it this way. To practice mindfulness in all of the ways recommended by the sutta would have been (and continues to be) a serious, time-consuming, and complex process involving not just calm attention to the breath but also engagement with sophisticated intellectual learning, emotionally evocative imagery, management of cognition and affect, and demanding moral commitments. It carves out a taxonomy that frames and guides the meditator's experience, suggesting what one should attend to and how one should attend to it. It suggests how to cultivate and sustain particular affective dispositions and intellectual ideas. It redefines practitioners' very sense of selfhood, first, by helping redefine their identities not as householders with family and caste lineages but as monastics, with different ways of being, seeing, speaking, and acting; and second by dismantling one's very sense of being a unitary, enduring self and replacing it with five component processes. Mindfulness on the model of the SP, therefore, is a highly constructive, imaginative, goal-oriented, conceptually and emotionally engaged enterprise.

Meditative insight—seeing things "as they are"—as presented in the SP and related texts, is not simply matter of bare, nonjudgmental, nonconceptual attention to the present moment, nor does it obviously yield an unmediated, objective knowledge stripped of all cultural conditioning. Rather, it is a more complex and culturally embedded affair that entails constructing an alternative system of concepts, forming alternative dispositions, creating different bases of valuing, and reconditioning—not just deconditioning—habits of mind and body. The meditative traditions in Pali Buddhism aim to produce new forms of ethical subjectivity in the sense that they provide exercises by which one comes to inhabit the norms and values of the tradition. One unlearns certain habitual emotions, desires, bodily activities supplied by the normative social imaginary and learns other ways of framing the world conceptually, of valuing certain things and devaluing others, of training the emotions, of dwelling in the categories supplied by the Buddhist tradition. It involves using the imagination to reconfigure one's interiority, learning to pay attention to particular aspects of experience, be watchful of the states of mind given in the tradition, fostering motivations encouraged by the tradition and curbing those it condemns. Ancient meditators acquired new sensibilities through training their bodies, senses, ideas, perceptions, emotions, and habits. They learned to feel disgust rather than desire for bodies; they learned to watch for rapture; they learned to move in dignified, controlled ways—and all of this eventually, if pursued with diligence, became naturalized.[5]

The fact that the meditative path we have been describing was deeply embedded in ancient Indian monastic life does not mean, however, that these practices cannot take on new significance and meaning in other contexts. In fact, they have been reinterpreted and recontextualized many times before they ever reached Europe and the Americas. Today's Standard Version of mindfulness meditation inherited several elements from the SP: attention to the breath as a calming and focusing device, careful observation of thought and feeling, and contemplation of the body (albeit, radically reinterpreted as the "body scan"). Much of the rest of the text is filtered out in secularized meditation, as it is highly specific to the Buddhist tradition. We will examine some of underlying intellectual and cultural conditions that provided the filters—as well as the magnets that attracted these selected elements—in subsequent chapters. Another element that contemporary meditative practices have inherited is a basic dialectical tension between the processes of systematically dismantling accepted understandings, attitudes, and ways of being in the world and reconstructing alternative ones.

Again, my intention in comparing and contrasting these contexts is not to suggest that contemporary iterations of these practices are deficient (or, for that matter, better) in comparison with ancient ones, nor to insist that their formation is so deeply embedded in cultural contexts that they cannot be meaningfully practiced in modern ones. Instead, I want to suggest that some groundwork needs to take place in order to have these more evaluative conversations more productively. That groundwork involves excavating certain elements of the social imaginary in which these practices are nestled in order to examine how these practices function in those contexts. In the next chapter, I theorize this issue more thoroughly.

6

Meditation and Cultural Repertoires

Taxonomies, Symptoms, and Cultural Contexts

The SP and other Pali meditation texts complicate the popular picture of meditation and mindfulness as mainly a matter of relaxation and nonjudgmental, present-centered awareness. Or as a free-form, open-ended or "objective" observation of contents of consciousness analogous to the investigation of the natural world by scientists. Moreover, our discussion of meditation within particular social imaginaries complicates the view, implicit in many of the neuroscientific studies of meditation today, that meditation simply reproduces mental "states" that are the same across time and space. For over a century Buddhists, Buddhist sympathizers, and scholars have talked about meditation as a kind of empirical or scientific investigation of the mind. This suggests a picture of the mind as containing contents that are accessible to reflexive introspection. If we apply this idea to the SP, it suggests that meditation on the aggregates, for example, would amount to simply penetrating though the illusions of a fixed, permanent self to discover lying beneath it, five aggregates waiting to be apprehended. Or that when one meditates on the contents of consciousness that these contents are simply *there* as a raw, uninterpreted stream of events. Yet it is hard to make the case that we have the same access to the contents of consciousness as a scientist has to, say, the movements of molecules or the composition of rocks because of the constructive, imaginative, and cultural elements in play. If there is any realm in which the observer affects what is observed, it is consciousness. If we bracket the issue of the ontological truth of the aggregates and *dharmas*, we can understand them as constituting a model or portrait of the human being and its lifeworld—one that guides the cultivation of particular ways of being and understanding.

In contrast to the ontological view, then, let me offer an alternative one that attempts to theorize more adequately the role that cultural context plays in contemplative practices. I begin with perhaps an unlikely analogy: that of psychological—especially psychosomatic—illness, an illustration that I believe can be expanded to other kinds of experiences. Anthropological thinkers,

Rethinking Meditation. David L. McMahan, Oxford University Press. © Oxford University Press 2023.
DOI: 10.1093/oso/9780197661741.003.0006

cross-cultural psychologists, historians of medicine, and philosophers who study psychological illness in different cultural or historical settings have demonstrated that not only are the theoretical categories and explanations of psychological illness quite different across cultures and historical periods, but also that the symptoms themselves vary considerably. Take, for example, the widespread phenomenon of "hysterical paralysis" among upper-middle-class women in the nineteenth and early twentieth centuries. Today, the disorder is very uncommon (and differently understood), and we have a variety of new illnesses—ADHD, anorexia nervosa, borderline personality disorder, chronic fatigue syndrome, etc.—that appear to be, at least in part, products of particular cultural conditions. Medical historian Edward Shorter (1992) claims that each historical period (and by implication, cultural milieu) has its own "symptom pool" shaped in part by the available categories, templates, and models of illness established by the medical community itself and by the surrounding culture. Ethan Watters (2010), expanding on this point, suggests that psychosomatic illnesses in particular "are examples of the unconscious mind attempting to speak in a language of emotional distress that will be understood in its time" (32). Shorter argues that symptom pools emerge through a dynamic negotiation between the patient, the patient's unconscious, the doctor, and the broader culture:

> In psychosomatic illness, the body's response to stress or unhappiness is orchestrated by the unconscious. The unconscious mind, just like the conscious, is influenced by the surrounding culture, which has models of what it considers to be legitimate and illegitimate symptoms. . . . By defining certain symptoms as illegitimate, a culture strongly encourages patients not to develop them or to risk being thought "undeserving" individuals with no real medical problems. Accordingly there is great pressure on the unconscious mind to produce only legitimate symptoms. . . . [The unconscious mind] will strive to present symptoms that always seem, to the surrounding culture, legitimate evidence of organic disease. This striving introduces a historical dimension. As the culture changes its mind about what is legitimate disease and what is not, the pattern of psychosomatic illness changes. (1992, ix–x)

Patients, according to Shorter, present symptoms that accord with the medical diagnostics of their time and place—what he calls the "medical shaping of symptoms" (1). The authority of the doctor and the medical establishment is essential to this shaping, as are broader cultural and institutional realities like insurance companies and how they categorize illnesses and authorize treatment. Watters expands on the point, arguing that public recognition of a disease leads to people manifesting the behavior in order to seek help:

> Patients and doctors would then engage in what is called "illness negotiation," whereby they would together shape each other's perceptions of the behavior. In this negotiation the doctor would provide the scientific validation that the symptom was indeed indicative of a legitimate disease category, and new patients would increase the attention focused on the new symptom in the professional and popular press, creating a feedback loop that further established the legitimacy of the new symptom. (2010, 33)

This argument suggests something important not only about the historical contingency of the categorization of mental illness but also about illness itself: that at least some mental disturbance manifests in culturally available ways and that authoritative taxonomies penetrate the unconscious, structuring the illness itself. Some illnesses, no doubt, are physiologically based, but even these are mediated and interpreted through available categories. In Shorter's view, people have vague, undefined anxieties that manifest through a repertoire of available forms that are authenticated by the medical establishment's taxonomies of illnesses and symptoms.

If this is true of mental illness, then it makes sense that other modes of human life are similarly structured—including "symptoms" of mental health and human flourishing, meditative states, and religious experiences. Contemplative practices are modes of self-cultivation that strive to produce certain experiences, train the emotions and sensibilities, and cultivate certain virtues and ways of being in a world—a world that contains particular normative understandings of a good life, a holy life, a successful life, as well as conceptions of the person, the mind and its features, the potential for human development and cultivation, and various experiences that meditators will have at different stages on the path. In the early Buddhist example, the tradition supplies a view of the human being (the aggregates, sense capacities, etc.), moral and attitudinal valuations of various phenomena (the body, sexuality, sense objects), taxonomies of the many phenomena of the lived world (*dhammas*), and markers of progress in meditation (e.g., the progressively more rarified states of concentration [*jhānas*]). These provide ways of directing attention and navigating what is significant and insignificant in meditative practice. They provide guidance on fostering or constraining certain thoughts, feelings, emotional dispositions, and ethical motivations, and on developing valued skills and creating, disrupting, or perhaps transcending culturally available personal identities.

Various articulations of the Dharma contain complex maps of the lifeworld in a particular social imaginary, and these maps guide practitioners toward the goal of human life, identifying various important markers of progress and dangers along the way. This progress is not merely a matter of private mental states but is something worked out between individual practitioners, their teachers, the tradition, and the culture more broadly. Practitioners are always in a dialogue with all of these—dialogue in which the significance and meaning of their experiences are not only interpreted but also shaped. Like patients and their doctors, meditators often have intensive interactions with their teachers—we might think of it as "experience negotiation"—in which they attempt to discern the significance of their meditative experiences and interpret them according to the teachings (the Zen tradition of *dokusan* or *sanzen* is most notable here). Stages of the path found in texts, narratives of others' meditative experiences, teachers' instructions, and dharma talks are in a similar relationship to the practitioner as the relationship between a patient to physicians and authoritative maps of illness like the *Diagnostic and Statistical Manual of Mental Disorders.*

Most meditators have likely considered their maps to correspond to a preexisting architecture of the mind and reality; therefore, they have considerable incentive to interpret and produce experiences that conform to the map. Buddhist meditators, therefore, have striven to identify the markers of transition between the first *jhāna* (a concentrated state of rapture and pleasure with discursive thought) and the second (a state of rapture and pleasure *without* discursive thought) or to look for signs that they have attained "stream entry" (the condition of decisively entering the path to awakening). They have questioned basic intuitions, like that of a continuing, enduring self, and instead tried to isolate and identify the five aggregates in their own experience. In traditions that insist that all appearances are illusory, practitioners must train their minds to see the world itself as a kind of dream. In some traditions, they must try to imagine the world and themselves as having Buddha nature, perfect and already awakened, despite the ample evidence to the contrary. They must, in other words, reimagine themselves and the world in ways suggested by these maps, not only interpreting but also cultivating their experiences accordingly.

In this way, inchoate and unconscious impulses, impressions, and notions emerge into consciousness to take the shape of available categories in the tradition, the "always already" available ways of understanding. The various narratives of progress, maps of the path, models of enlightened persons, and instructions all constitute templates that shape how meditation works in configuring consciousness. These templates guide meditators toward attending to certain features of their experience, interpreting their significance, categorizing them in certain ways, acting on them according to prescribed purposes. And they may simply not notice what is not on a particular map. The many detailed maps of Buddhist paths—the *jhānas, lam rim, bhāvanākrama*, etc.— are in this view best seen as constructive models that do not simply represent a certain territory but configure it according to particular understandings of the Dharma. And if we recall again the SP, we can appreciate anew how little space it devotes to bare attention to the breath and how much to deeply internalizing the teachings and taxonomies of Buddhist doctrine by contemplating them in a concentrated, systematic way.

In order to appreciate something of the meaning, significance, and purpose of meditation in the earlier phases of Buddhism, we must take into account its initial status as a minority, world-renouncing, countercultural way of life. The general stance toward worldly phenomena in the Pali literature allows us to better understand the initial move of mindfulness of the body: "knowing that one is walking, etc.," i.e., the disruption of momentum of the habitual flow of activity through focused attention, particular to physical movements. First, this flow of activity is constituted by a pregiven social imaginary. This imaginary supplied a set of normative activities, an ensemble of cultural skills, a repertory of sensibilities, inclinations, concepts, and moral values to which anyone in this context would have been habituated. The monastic life was an alternative community that instilled different sensibilities, skills, attitudes, virtues, and values. Rather than valuing family, sexuality within marriage, prosperity, and a hopefully acquiring a satisfying life dodging misfortune through ritual activity and ingenuity, the monk (at least in theory) renounced all of these, left family, and was cautioned against longing to return to their love. He was taught that sensual and aesthetic pleasures were at best transitory and at worst imprisoning. He was strictly celibate, forbidden from making money and committed to poverty, and was taught that no amount of pleasing the gods, ritual action, or good luck could ever lead to a satisfying life in samsara.

To take these positions, especially in the early phases of Buddhism before it was well established, must have been difficult and controversial. Heavily conceptual and value-saturated meditation practices like those found in the SP served, therefore, not only to disrupt the culturally constituted unreflective flow of experience that took the values, sensibilities, and tacit assumptions of the dominant culture for granted, they also provided a new repertoire of values, attitudes, and ontological categories. But not only this: these contemplations were a way not just of supplying the alternative worldview of the Buddhadharma but also of deeply infusing it into lived experience—back into the tacit dimension—thereby reconfiguring it and transforming experience at the everyday level. Conceptual meditations were a way of re-envisioning the world, imparting an alternative framework, and reconfiguring not only explicit beliefs but also the more tacit, deep-seated orientations so that the Dharma would become naturalized. Such practices helped create and maintain an alternative social imaginary.

Two Meditators Again

With all of this in mind, let's try to imagine again our ancient Indian monk and our contemporary Vipassana practitioner from chapter 3 attempting to put some aspects of the SP into practice. As he sits down to focus on his breath, the monk attempts to disregard fond memories of his premonastic identity, his caste position, his sense of belonging to a particular clan and family, the physical comforts of home, and the emotional comforts of parents and siblings. He struggles to examine and release his ordinary sense of being an "I," with specific fixed characteristics. Instead he focuses on trying to identify the five processes he has been told he really is, the aggregates. Here is the body, but how to differentiate this present sense of the body (*rūpa*) from *feeling* (*vedanā*)? Is *this* a feeling or a perception (*sañña*)? Is the twinge of desire to give up on monastic life and return home a volition (*saṅkhāra*)? He suspects his mind is beginning to get caught in one of the five hindrances—restless worry—and attempts to let it go and replace it with serenity. A sexually charged image arises, and he displaces it with an image of a corpse in the cremation ground. He remembers the vivid portrayal of hell realms his teacher described and feels longing for the realm of the gods, where one lives for thousands of years without pain. He remembers that he should not be content, however, with aspiring to this realm and tries to form an image of the true goal, nirvana, beyond time and space, beyond even existence and nonexistence. Frustrated by the attempt, he recognizes that his mind is in a stream of conceptual rumination (*papañca*) and returns to the breath with a lingering image of the vast undifferentiated space of nirvana.

In this focused, effortful process, the monk is recreating himself in particular ways; he is shifting his sense of himself as he disregards certain aspects of his experience as illusory and cultivates others as true. He is alert to the subtle movements of his body, thought, and emotions, interpreting their significance according to the categories that he has been taught. His sense of subjectivity eventually becomes reconfigured based on his reimagining of himself as five aggregates rather than a permanent self. He must manage his desires as well, steering them away from sensual pleasures and even from the pleasures of the *deva* realm to the more abstract goal of nirvana.

And what about our contemporary meditator? She sits down and calms her mind, trying to bring to attention her deepest aspirations. She has been told to acknowledge all thoughts and feelings and let them go, not judging them, repressing them, clinging to them, or letting them proliferate into an internal conversation. Yet when an angry thought emerges toward a colleague at work, she cannot help judging it unworthy of her spiritual aspirations, and she has to force her mind back to her breath to avoid developing an imaginary and heated conversation with the colleague. When a wave of well-being sweeps over her, she identifies *that* as more of what she is after, then calls this into question, remembering her instructions to just observe thoughts and feelings and not prefer one to another. This is followed by a memory of her brother, who is having trouble with his marriage. She is briefly angry with him, but then a small eruption of love arises—no matter what he has done to complicate his life, she accepts him. *That*, she guesses, may be the unconditional loving-kindness that she should feel toward him described by the Pali term, *metta*. Maybe it is even the unconditioned love she recently read about in a modern Tibetan teacher's book, a love that dwells in each of us and is our fundamental nature, waiting to be discovered. She tries to remember if there is anything like this idea in the *vipassanā* books she has read, then refocuses on her breathing, trying to put away all of these speculations. At some point her mind becomes focused so that she is continuously attending to her breath as it streams in and out of her body. Thoughts, feelings, and sensations arise but dissipate before taking root in ongoing narratives. As a peaceful feeling permeates her body, she briefly wonders if her amygdala has become less active and if blood is flowing freely to her parietal lobes. She is pleased that her meditation may be creating new neural connections that will allow her to think more clearly, pay closer attention, and be more compassionate. After a few more minutes of calm focus on her breath, her electronic bell rings, and she is off to work, trying to maintain a sense of calm and clarity, feeling better about how she might interact with her colleague.

By some accounts this might be considered a rather superficial meditation. Some might say that she only was really meditating in the last few minutes when her mind became calm and focused. But there is, nevertheless, a practice of self-cultivation doing its work throughout. She attends to certain aspects of her experience rather than others; she imagines herself in certain ways according to dominant scientific theories; she envisions certain ends she wants to achieve through her practice. She struggles to reconcile different strands of thinking in different Buddhist traditions, to reconcile *doing* with *not-doing*, to reconcile trying to actualize certain states of mind, moral intuitions, aesthetic sensibilities with allowing whatever emerges to emerge without judgment or interference. In judging her thoughts and feelings, trying not to judge them, subtly choosing to try to foster compassion rather than resentment, noticing anger, struggling to identify what might be a hidden and more profound level of her own being, she is cultivating herself using several interlacing taxonomies—Buddhist, therapeutic, neuroscientific—all taking place in the wider, more tacit and unconscious structures of life within her social imaginary. All of this even when she is being asked to *just sit*.

We should take care again to emphasize the point that in engaging in a playful act of imagining two meditators in very different contexts, we are not presenting a simple East-versus-West, ancient-versus-modern, or, even less, an authentic-versus-inauthentic dichotomy and thereby suggesting that "the twain shall never meet." I am emphasizing specific areas of contrast in two different social imaginaries in order to demonstrate that context matters. Are the modern professional and the ancient monk doing something utterly different? Certainly there is overlap: both follow their breath, calm their minds and bodies, try to cultivate compassion and avoid hatred, greed, and ignorance. But the familial, institutional, social, cultural, civilizational, and cosmic contexts in which they enact these values could hardly be more divergent. The modern professional has a family to which she is deeply committed, a job that sustains her, arts and entertainment, and broader commitments to gender equality, human rights, individual choice, and many other nonnegotiable goods. She lives, in other words, in an entirely different social imaginary with different default intuitions and a different repertoire of possible ways of being than the ancient monk. Some of the things that mindfulness helps her with are expressly forbidden the monk: parenting, money-making, love-making, play-watching. So mindfulness and meditation can help to cultivate very different kind of people. Clearly these are flexible practices that have been adapted today to quite different ends within disparate lived worlds.

That the meaning, significance, and purpose of contemplative practices, or any other human activity, would be deeply shaped by their social context is obvious for anyone in the humanities and social sciences. The point I am arguing, however, goes a bit further. It asserts that meditation "works" as a systemic part of the ecology of a sociocultural system. It may be used to cultivate available ways of being in a given culture, to challenge them, or to create alternative ones; but it cannot operate in a vacuum. Even if it is stripped of much of its earlier contexts—as it has in some contemporary situations—then, like a dry sponge, it absorbs culturally available ideas, values, and aspirations, which provide a structure in which the practices become meaningful in new ways.

This must challenge any account of how meditation works simply in terms of universal states of mind, be they articulated either in the normative terms of tradition or in modern scientific terms.[1]

And Yet . . .

Despite all of the points I have just argued, there is, I now must confess, something incomplete about this picture. No doubt it will have occurred to many familiar with Buddhist traditions that part of their genius is that they themselves have recognized the constructed nature of all maps and models, templates and taxonomies—even Buddhist ones. The Buddhist understanding that all categories are conceptual constructions is based more on linguistic and philosophical considerations than observations about culture and history—the latter seem to be a mostly modern insight—nevertheless, it is undeniable. Indeed, one of the fundamental creative tensions in and between Buddhist traditions has been between what I have been calling their *constructive* and *deconstructive* aspects. I have so far offered a mostly constructivist approach to meditation, in which people attempt to actualize particular ways of being laid out by authoritative texts and teachings (be they suttas or psychotherapists) within the taxonomies, possibilities, and limitations of particular traditions and social imaginaries. This entails not only conscious effort to *be* certain ways—compassionate, insightful, calm—but also unconscious processes that guide the mind to actualize ideals of the tradition and the culture laid out in various maps, models, and templates.

I have presented this process as reliant on the authority of tradition, texts, and teachers, which make these ways of being, rooted in the available taxonomies and forms of life in a particular social imaginary, appear uniquely real and natural, based on the authority of enlightened beings. This cannot help but seem to put me, the scholar *qua* scholar, in a position of appearing to know something the practitioner does not know—that these taxonomies and forms of life are contingent constructions, not built in to reality itself. But the tradition itself winds back around to tap me on the shoulder. Buddhist philosophers have often asserted the constructedness of their own categories and taxonomies and have worked in sophisticated and creative ways to explore the issue. Perfection of Wisdom literature, for example, plays with the tradition's sacred conceptions, positing them, then gleefully dismantling them, challenging readers to find solid conceptual ground to stand on and insisting there is none, taking the reader to the very boundaries of propositional language in order to reveal the shimmering fragility of all categories.

Some Zen literature takes this deconstructive route to the extreme, inverting cherished binary oppositions—purity and impurity, *saṃsāra* and nirvana—sweeping away taxonomies, tearing up the scriptures, killing the Buddha. Consider the words attributed to Bodhidharma, the legendary founder of Chan: "Trying to find a Buddha or enlightenment is like trying to grab space. Space has a name but no form. It's not something you can pick up or put down. And you certainly can't grab it. Beyond this mind you'll never see a Buddha. The Buddha is a product of your mind. Why look for a Buddha beyond this mind?" (Bodhidharma 1987, 9–10). Even in early Buddhist meditation traditions, it is possible to argue that all of the reshaping of cognition and affect is meant to be preparatory for a more radical dissolution of all constructed states of consciousness.[2] Indeed, many philosophical debates between Buddhist schools have been about where to draw the line between what is fabricated by consciousness and what (if anything) is not.

So in the next chapter, we must give some sense of the other side of the picture and discuss some examples of deconstructive meditation, in which the practitioner is to recognize the fabricated nature of all concepts, as well as meditations that posit an original Buddha-nature in everyone—therefore, there is precisely nothing that needs to be done: no cultivation of virtues, no rigorous discipline, no precise comportment. Just be what you are, find the Buddha within you. If this is sounding closer to modern articulations of meditation, it is because this approach too, mainly derived from Zen traditions, is a crucial factor in the lineage of contemporary versions of mindfulness.

7

Deconstructive Meditation and the Search for the Buddha Within

Dispatches from the Worlds of Meditation: 7

The emptiness of the mind is something we can "see," so to speak. When we look at the mind, it's like infinite space. It has no limit. It has no material form, color, or shape. There is nothing we can touch. That space, that openness, is the empty nature of our mind. When contemplating mind's emptiness, experience the spacious, insubstantial, nonmaterial quality of mind, of thoughts and emotions, and leave the mind in a state of ease and total openness.

—Dzogchen Ponlop Rinpoche[1]

The Dharma Game: Categories and the Way Things Are

When introducing the Buddhist idea of *dharmas* to my college students, we play what I have come to call the "dharma game."[2] Dharma is an extremely polyvalent word in South Asian literature, but in this specialized, philosophical sense it refers the basic, fundamental elements of existence or the building blocks of experience. They can be physical factors, like form or shape (*rūpa*) or mental factors like attention, hatred, or analysis. Any particular combination of these basic building blocks makes up a moment of experience and is causally constituted by previous combinations of dharmas. We can think of them as the basic constituents of the lifeworld. Before even talking about dharmas in Buddhism, though, I ask students to come up with a list of basic categories that might qualify as fundamental elements of human experience. I start them off with "vision," after which they quickly fill in the remaining five senses—hearing, smelling, and so on. Then they piece together other contenders. Someone might offer, for example, "emotion," after which others will try to determine the basic, fundamental human emotions. Most agree that "love"

Rethinking Meditation. David L. McMahan, Oxford University Press. © Oxford University Press 2023.
DOI: 10.1093/oso/9780197661741.003.0007

and "hatred" and "disgust" qualify, but by the time they get to something like jealousy or embarrassment, they are less sure that these are fundamental or derivative of some more basic emotion. We might discuss whether some emotions might be specific to a particular culture or age, like "fomo"—fear of missing out—which seems dependent on, or at least exacerbated by, ubiquitous social media. Other candidates for fundamental elements of experience emerge, like anxiety, attention, anticipation, doubt. Some more philosophically astute students might zero in on things like being in three-dimensional space, experiencing the flow of time, the use of language, or the ability to reflect on one's mortality.

After a while we have thirty or forty terms on the board. Then I show them some charts of dharmas as conceived in the Abhidharma literature, the early Buddhist literature that attempted to organize and interpret the teachings of the Buddha into a coherent, consistent, and systematic philosophy. First we look at a chart of seventy-five dharmas from the Sarvāstivāda school of Indian Buddhism.

The Seventy-Five Dharmas According to the Sarvāstivāda Abhidharma

I. Conditioned (*saṃskṛta*)
   A. Form (*rūpa*)
      i. visual awareness, auditory awareness, olfactory awareness, flavor-awareness, tactile awareness; objects of vision, sound, smell, taste, touch; nonmaterial forms
   B. Consciousness (*citta*)
   C. Mental factors (*caitasika*)
      i. General faculties (*mahābhūmika*)
         - feeling, volition, perception, inclination, contact, understanding, mindfulness, attention, determination, concentration
      ii. Virtuous qualities (*kuśala*)
         - conviction, diligence, calm, equanimity, modesty, shame, absence of greed, absence of hatred, absence of violence, vigor
      iii. Mental afflictions (*kleśa*)
         - delusion, lack of diligence, lethargy, lack of conviction, torpor, restlessness
      iv. Nonvirtuous qualities (*akuśala*)
         - nonmodesty, shamelessness
      v. Impurities (*parīttakleśa*)
         - anger, enmity, dishonesty, jealousy, spite, concealment, avarice, deceptiveness, pride, harmfulness

   vi. Indeterminate dharmas (*aniyata*)
       – remorse, sleep, reasoning, investigation, greed, hostility, conceit, doubt
   D. Conditioned dharmas without thought (*cittaviprayukta saṃskāra*)
       i. acquisition, nonacquisition, similarity, lack of ideation, ideationless attainment, attainment of cessation, vital faculty, production, subsistence, deterioration, impermanence, words, phrases, syllables
2. Unconditioned dharmas (*asaṃskṛta*)
   A. space, cessation through reflection, cessation without reflection[3]

We consider how many of the terms on the chart overlap with those the students generated. Some do, but others seem rooted in particularly Buddhist ways of understanding things. Mindfulness, for example, is considered to be a dharma, as are equanimity and nonattachment. "Similarity" or "subsistence" seldom occur to students as fundamental building blocks of experience. The discrepancies between our off-the-cuff chart and the Abhidharma chart begin to open up a hint of skepticism about the prospects for the entire project, for if we are trying to come up with the basic components of human experience, then these should, of course, be true for all humans no matter when and where they lived. This conviction certainly seems implicit in the project of the Abhidharma philosophers, as well as cognitive scientists who might ask similar questions today. Cultural relativity rears its head, casting doubt that one can, in fact, acquire an all-encompassing, culture-neutral view of the matter.

The problem is exacerbated when I show another chart, this one from the Yogācāra school of Buddhism, which insists that there are, in fact, not seventy-five but rather one hundred dharmas. They add categories like "speed" (*java*) (one might think contemporary people would have come up with this one!) and "holding a view as supreme" (considered an "affliction"). Now the problem becomes more complicated. Whenever anyone tries to come to a definitive theoretical account of human experience, much less a definitive *number* of its basic constituents, there is certain to be disagreement. Once you have a number, whether it's 75, 100, or 82 (the number in the Theravāda school), someone is bound to insist that you missed one or that you included one that shouldn't be included. Appealing to the Buddha doesn't help. In the early discourses attributed to the Buddha, he doesn't weigh in on the subject; indeed, such systematization of the Buddha's teachings in the Abhidharma texts were in part an attempt to nail down things left ambiguous in the earlier literature. The lack of agreement, even among supposedly enlightened scholars, invites the paradox of conceptual *constructedness*, that is, the fact that any attempt to establish the final theoretical shape of reality irrespective of human conceptual constructions begins to look very much like a construction itself. Perhaps meditation rather than scholasticism might resolve the issue? Not likely, since meditators seem to have come to no more universal agreement than philosophers.

We've seen in the last chapter that different social imaginaries, and different systems of thought within these imaginaries, have different taxonomies of experience. The Abhidharma literature of various Buddhist schools established several. Modern medicine has one too, and these systems are not only different ways of carving up the world of human experience but also, in some measure, of constituting it. Yet, we should not think that Buddhists were simply and naïvely trapped in these systems. In fact, some classical Buddhist thinkers wrestled with questions similar to those that modern thinkers have asked in different ways: if we are always embedded in social, linguistic, cultural contexts, how do we step back and "see" those contexts if they are like the water in which the fish swims? Is it possible to get outside of one's system of concepts and categories—one's social imaginary—or does it determine everything one can think (including the desire to get out of it)? Can we transcend our culturally specific ways of thinking, feeling, and being? Can we make definitive statements about things "as they are"?

Emptiness and the Way Things Are

Our way of making arguments like this today often hinges on cultural or historical difference—people in different times and places with different languages and conceptual repertoires may see and feel things differently. Early Buddhists seemed to recognize this issue too. In the *Assalayana Sutta* (M ii 147), the Buddha makes an argument for a kind of cultural relativism against a young Brahmin's insistence that, among the four social classes (*varṇa*), only the Brahmins can be spiritually purified. The Buddha responds by noting that, while there are indeed four classes where they live, in a nearby area there is a society with only two classes, and they sometimes change places. The obvious implication: the division of human beings into four categories is not built into the nature of things but is merely a product of arbitrary, local social arrangements. The idea of one class being inherently pure and others not, therefore, makes no sense.

In Buddhist philosophy, these questions were more often examined not through the lens of cultural difference, however, but through the recognition of the constructive powers of language and concepts. Around the turn of the first millennium, such considerations began to call into question the entire scholastic project of coming up with a definitive account of the fundamental constituents of experience, the dharmas, and to invite a backlash, a kind of antitheory, that attempted to push the entire effort to its limits and go beyond it. The Perfection of Wisdom literature, along with the Madhyamaka school of Mahāyāna Buddhism, supplied the method for the endeavor: a revision of the concept of emptiness (*śūnyatā*). A great deal has been written on emptiness, and we only need give a basic summary here in order to think through some implications for meditation.[4] In emptiness philosophy, nothing has inherent existence (*svabhāva*) or an intrinsic, independent, and permanent nature. Instead, everything is in process and dependent on other things, that is, *empty* of, or lacking, its own fixed, independent being. Abhidharma thought asserted that, while this was true of things like chairs and people, the dharmas were fundamental entities, the essential elements of existence out of which everything in the perceived world was constituted. Emptiness philosophy insisted that even dharmas were empty; there are no unchanging constituents (as the Sarvāstivāda school insisted the dharmas were) but only shifting patterns with no permanent, substantial ontological substrate. This means that all categories are constituted by language, concepts, and conventions; our words and concepts do not simply correspond to independent realities but, rather, they carve up and constitute the lived world in particular ways. Everything that is thinkable and sayable is relative and conventional, which eliminates the possibility of a final, correct taxonomy or an absolutely correct philosophical "view" (*dṛṣṭi*).

The critique of dharma theory from the perspective of emptiness shifted, in some texts, the object of meditative inquiry. Recall that the approach to meditation in some contexts was to analyze conceptual constructions into their component parts, thus deconstructing the ordinary boundaries between things into more fundamental ones—the dharmas. Meditation under the influence of emptiness philosophy targets the dharmas themselves for deconstruction. For example, rather than identifying particular dharmas as virtuous or nonvirtuous, the goal was to see through these distinctions to the more fundamental constructedness of all phenomena. Even these supposedly fundamental constituents of experience were relative phenomena constituted by concepts and conventions. The goal of meditation on this model, then, becomes achieving this *one* insight: the lack of fixed, permanent, independent nature in everything. The Perfection of Wisdom literature illustrates this attempt to undermine the idea that the dharmas—or anything else—constitute a fixed, underlying architecture of reality:

Foolish, undeveloped, common people settle down in all of the dharmas. Having (conceptually) constructed them, attached to the binary oppositions (of either independent existence or non-existence), they do not know or see those dharmas. So they construct dharmas that are not really found. . . . After constructing them, they settled down in name and form . . . and don't know or see the path that truly is. (*Aṣṭa*, 15)

But if the dharmas are not fundamental realities, what *is* the reality of things? One way this text puts it is that everything is *ananta*—unending, boundless, infinite. "Every being is endless and boundless because one cannot get at its beginning, middle, and end" (*Aṣṭa*, 49). That is, every taxonomy carves up reality in a particular way, drawing lines around things, distinguishing them from other things, and the "things" themselves are constituted by this activity, not by something they are in and of themselves. This construction of "things" helps us get around in the world on a practical basis. There is nothing inherent in a red, hexagonal metal plate with white lines that naturally commands one to stop. Yet, according to convention, when driving we stop at a stop sign (and we should!). This is what Nāgārjuna, the second-century philosopher, called "conventional truth" (*saṃvṛti-sātya*). At a conventional level, we can distinguish between stop signs and other traffic signs. And, importantly, we can make legitimate distinctions within the realm of conventional truth. Just because everything is empty of a fixed, essential nature doesn't mean that we can arbitrarily decide that a stop sign means "go," or "take off your shoes." There is conventional truth *and* falsehood. And yet, ultimately, everything that we can designate in some way is a conventional rather than absolute reality, not just street signs but all things. Nor does it mean that things do not really exist at all and are mere hallucinations (though some emptiness literature does lean in this direction). Rather, it is that the emergence in the lifeworld of any individual phenomenon comes about both through past causes and conditions and through its delineation by language, concepts, and conventions rather than through its own inherent, independent nature.

A particular wristwatch can be delineated from all other things. Yet it is not an independent, permanent entity. It is constituted by the materials that have been in the earth for millions of years; by the fact that we have conventions of measuring time in particular units—hours and minutes—that we represent by two moving bars on a circular surface; that someone had the idea for the design of this specific watch; that particular people showed up at the watch factory the day it was made. At some point it will cease to be a functioning watch, it will disintegrate, and all of its materials will go on to become other things. In the torrent of all of these causes and conditions, in the history of materials coming together and falling apart, it is we who draw the line around "watch" and delimit it, for a time, from all other objects. It is likewise, according to Madhyamaka thought, with all things, including even the most basic, seemingly elementary ones like the dharmas. Everything emerges in dependence on countless causes and conditions, and fixing any object as a permanent, independent, and enduring thing is an illusion. It is in this sense that the Perfection of Wisdom says that there is "no beginning, middle, and end" to anything. Everything is boundless—that is, without a purely natural boundary between one thing and another. Such boundaries and distinctions are a function of the mind. Philosophers and ordinary people alike, however, tend toward *reification* (*satyābhimāna*; Tib. *bden 'dzin*) of the objects of mind, that is, taking these conceptual designations as independently real entities. Deeply understanding that everything lacks an independent, inherent existence, and thus is boundless, becomes the goal of meditation in some Mahāyāna formulations, and doing so entails *dereifying* these conceptual designations.

Thus we find in the voluminous *Perfection of Wisdom in 100,000 Lines* a strange chapter. It consists of a version of the *Sutta on the Foundations of Mindfulness* (SP) quite similar to the one we have discussed, but with an uncanny difference. At the end of each set of instructions, the text essentially says that everything meditators are instructed to do in the various contemplations, any states they attempt to produce or eliminate, virtues they try to actualize, the very Eightfold Path that they attempt to follow are to be understood through "nonapprehension" (*anupalabdha*) of an inherent, independent, permanent existence; that is seeing them all as empty (*śūnya*).

> Here a Bodhisattva knows, when he walks, "I walk," when he stands, "I stand," when he sits, "I sit," when he lies down, "I lie down." In whichever position his body may be placed, whether in a good way or not, he knows that it is in that position. And that through nonapprehension (of anything). (Conze 1975, 153)

All of the categories enumerated in the original SP are enumerated here; however, the essential insight proposed in this version is that they are all conceptual constructs and have no inherent, independent reality. And that is the one insight that the meditator needs to acquire. All of the states, attitudes, virtues, and values that the previous meditation literature suggests cultivating, and all of the faults, hindrances, and afflictive states that one should eschew, ultimately lack any inherent existence. Thus they should not be "apprehended" as such. The dharma game is over.

Beyond Categories

Let's take a step back for a moment. The argument I have been making, recall, is that meditative practices are means of cultivating particular ways of being in the world, that these ways of being occur in particular social contexts with repertoires of culturally available ideas, ideals, attitudes, ethical orientations, and default intuitions. In this sense, these practices are not simply means of cutting off socially constructed conceptions and getting to an unmediated truth within the private, individual mind; rather, they create conditions for alternative conceptual constructions, attitudes, and ways of being. These ways are also constituted, at least in part, by culturally available categories, though they may create ruptures in a given social imaginary to catalyze something novel—a new conception of how to be, what reality is, or what the self is.

This analysis is rooted in modern humanistic and social thought. As I hinted at the end of the last chapter, though, Buddhist thought itself has come to parallel conclusions, i.e., that the world of human experience is constructed by our linguistic and conceptually constructed categories. Moreover, it affirms, it is possible to see these categories *as* constructions and to penetrate through them, either to something more real or to a blissful freedom from being constrained by them. For the Abhidharma literature, the "more real" that meditation reveals is the dharmas, a set of basic building blocks of the lived world. Mahāyāna thought begins to experiment with pushing deconstructive analysis to the dharmas themselves, declaring even these supposed basic constituents to be linguistic and conceptual fabrications— relative, conventional truths (*saṃvṛti-sātya*), rather than truth in the highest sense (*paramārthya-sātya*). The dilemma of emptiness is that it pushes *unconstructed* truth to something so elusive that it cannot be found, thought, or conceptualized. If even the supposedly unconstructed dharmas—nirvana, space—are actually conceptual constructs themselves, truth in the highest sense is an ever-receding horizon, impossible to pin down—and yet, according to the tradition, possible to realize by releasing all "pinning down."

In the Perfection of Wisdom literature, those who understand this are bodhisattvas, who are free from getting entrapped in any conceptual configuration or taxonomy of categories—even Buddhist ones. They are able to tolerate the fear of realizing that everything is empty and that there is no solid ground to existence. Even wisdom and enlightenment, as concepts, seem to get swept away. Indeed, the concept of emptiness itself is empty! Discussions of this bring referential language to its limits.

No wisdom can we get hold of, no highest perfection,
No Bodhisattva, no thought of enlightenment either.
When told of this, not bewildered and in no way anxious,
A Bodhisattva courses in the Well-Gone's [Buddha's] wisdom.
In form, in feeling, will, perception and awareness
Nowhere in them they find a place to rest on.
Without a home they wander, dharmas never hold them,
Nor do they grasp at them . . . . (Conze 1973, 9)

Not grasping at dharmas, avoiding their reification, includes not grasping even at Buddhist teachings as if they are final endpoints in analysis or ultimate statements of truth. Everything asserted is in scare quotes. Thus the shocking verses in the *Heart Sūtra* that insist that from the perspective of emptiness none of the settled categories of even the Buddhist tradition—including the Four Truths and the Eightfold Path—have any ultimate reality:

With regard to emptiness, there is no form, no feeling, no perception, no volition, no consciousness; no eye, ear, nose, tongue, body, mind; no form, sound, smell, taste, touch, or objects of mind; no ignorance, no ending of ignorance . . . no old age and death, no ending of old age and death. There is no suffering, no origination, no cessation, no path.

While the Pali version of the SP suggested that the practitioner contemplate and internalize the various categories of Buddhist thought—make them real in one's experience—this passage suggests contemplating the emptiness of these categories, the fact that they are merely conventional truths. This approach pulls the rug of any concepts, images, ideals, and values out from beneath one's feet and leaves a vertiginous sense of being suspended in space. (Indeed, unobstructed space [ākāśa] is a common metaphor for the mind that has realized emptiness.) Emptiness literature admits that this can be a fearful place to be, one that might lead one to nihilism or terror at things suddenly being deprived of the sense of reality. A "wrongly grasped emptiness," as Nāgārjuna puts it, is like a snake grabbed from the wrong end—it can come back to bite you. And yet this dereification is not mere blankness. Truth in the highest sense exists; it just cannot be put in any formulation or "view." It is described as a blissful, liberating realization. All that has seemed an obstacle, a hindrance, or a weight is dissolved. And so the *Heart Sūtra* avows: "The bodhisattva, relying on the Perfection of Wisdom, dwells without obstacles of thought. Without obstacles of thought, he does not tremble, he has overcome fear, and he attains nirvana." In some texts, people weep and dance with joy upon realizing emptiness.

Meditation and the Buddha Within

Another closely related element in Mahāyāna reformulations of meditation is what John Dunne has aptly called "innateist" forms of meditation. Dunne points out that, by the third century or so, there is a spectrum in Buddhist thought between the *constructivist* approach—which asserts that progress toward awakening is acquired gradually through both eliminating obstructions and cultivating the characteristics and virtues of a buddha—and the *innateist* approach—which insists that buddhahood is innate in everyone (Dunne 2011). On the former model, one must cultivate or construct the qualities and virtues of a buddha, little-by-little, perhaps over many lifetimes. On the latter model, all of the qualities of a buddha—buddha-nature—are inherent within every living being. Some East Asian thinkers extend this even to inanimate objects and all of the cosmos.

Among the proponents of the doctrine of buddha-nature, there exists another spectrum: between those who assert that everyone has the *potential* to become a buddha and those who argue, more radically, that everyone is *already* a buddha, but their awakened nature is obscured by adventitious mental impurities. As the Buddha in the *Tathāgata-garbha Sūtra* puts it: "All beings, though they find themselves with all sorts of kleshas [defilements, mental impurities], have a tathagata-garbha [matrix or womb of the Buddha] that is eternally unsullied, and that is replete with virtues no different from my own" (Grosnick 1995, 96).[5] The *Tathāgata-garbha Sūtra* insists that you should "not consider yourselves inferior or base. You all personally possess the [buddha-nature]." Nevertheless, you must "exert yourselves and destroy your past evils" and clear away afflictive mental states in order to reveal the buddha within (Grosnick, 101). If buddhahood is present in people only in potential, practitioners must nurture the seeds of buddhahood by developing understanding, ethical activity, and meditative wisdom. The idea that it is innate, fully developed but hidden deep within, would have important implications on how meditation was conceived in some traditions.

Some of the formative literature of the Chan/Zen tradition radically rethinks meditative practice in light of the idea that all beings are already buddhas but just don't realize it. In the *Platform Sutra of the Sixth Patriarch*, for example, Huineng declares that meditation should not be conceived as giving rise to wisdom, for beings are already wise buddhas. Meditation does not cultivate or create virtues or even clear off "dust" from the mirror of the mind. Dust and mirror are all one in buddha-nature. The point of sitting in meditation becomes, therefore, the stilling of conceptual formations and attachments in order to let the innate buddha-nature shine through (McRae 2000).

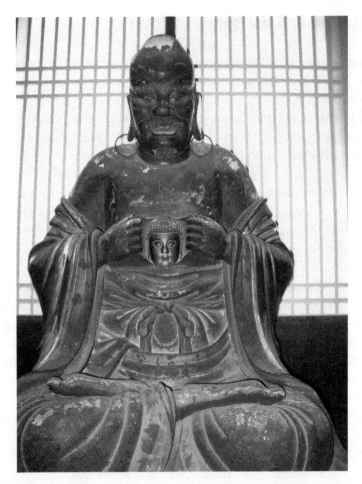

FIGURE 7.1 The Arhat Rāhula (*Ragora Sonja*), from Eighteen Arhats (*Rakan*), by Fan Daosheng (Han Dōsei, 1635–1670). Manpuku-ji Temple, Kyoto. Photo by Eric Greene.

In a similar vein, according to the ninth-century Chan master, Huangbo:

The Buddhas and all the sentient beings are only the One Mind—there are no other dharmas. . . . It transcends all limitations, names, traces, and correlations. It in itself—that's it! To activate thoughts is to go against it! It is like space, which is boundless and immeasurable.

It is only this One Mind that is Buddha; there is no distinction between Buddhas and sentient beings. However, sentient beings are attached to characteristics and seek outside themselves. Seeking it, they lose it even more. Sending the Buddha in search of the Buddha, grasping the mind with the mind, they may exhaust themselves in striving for an entire eon but will never get it. They do not understand that if they cease their thoughts and end their thinking, the Buddha will automatically be present. . . .

    This mind is the Buddha; the Buddha is the sentient being. When it is sentient being, the mind is not lessened; and when it is [one of] the Buddhas, the mind is not increased. And as for the six perfections (pāramitās) and the myriad practices, and the types of merit as numerous as the [sands of the] Ganges River—[every sentient being is] fundamentally sufficient in these and requires no further cultivation. (McRae: 2005, 13)

The goal of meditation here—if it is appropriate even to assert a goal—is not the cultivation of the many characteristics of a buddha but the realization that one is already a buddha. In this sense, "thinking"—or at least becoming attached to one's thoughts and reifying them—becomes an obstacle to perceiving one's true nature as a buddha.

    This style of meditation in the innateist strains of the Mahāyāna, especially Zen, is an important source of the emphasis in contemporary mindfulness on not thinking, not judging, and staying in the present moment. Dunne offers a parallel example of the style from the Tibetan Mahāmudrā tradition found in the ninth Karmapa, Wangchûg Dorjé's sixteenth-century text, *The Ocean of Definitive Meaning*. In one set of instructions, Dorjé directs readers not to attempt to actualize certain experiences and avoid others, as the classical meditation literature advises. Instead, he instructs them to release all seeking and rest in the present moment:

Thus, do not give your mind work to do. Let it go, and without meditating on anything, rest it in a relaxed, open and clear way in a state of mere nondistraction without making any adjustments at all. Relax openly into a state without expectations or judgments. In that state, do not chase the past, do not invite the future. Place awareness in the present without correction or expectation. (Dunne 2015, 264)

The Japanese Zen master Dōgen (1200–1253) offers a similar approach in his instructions on seated meditation (*zazen*): "Cast aside all involvements and discontinue all affairs. Do not think of good or evil; do not deal with right or wrong. Halt the revolutions of the mind, intellect, and consciousness; stop the calculations of thought, ideas, and perceptions" (Bielefeldt 1988, 177).

    There are, of course, significant differences between these disparate Chinese, Japanese, and Tibetan practices; however, they share a general approach to meditation: attempting to still the mind of conceptual thought, avoiding dwelling in the past or anticipating the future, eschewing attempts to subdue destructive states of mind or encourage favorable ones, and refraining from steering the mind toward any goal except that of maintaining undistracted attention on the present experience, whatever it may be. Moreover, the underlying rationale is the same in these innateist practices: the clearing away of cognitive and affective obscurations to reveal one's innate buddha-nature.

In some literature, this approach might seem to entail a strain of iconoclasm, and even a disregard for ethical standards, the strict discipline of a monk—and even meditation itself. For example, Linji, the ninth-century founder of the Linji (Jpn: Rinzai) school of Chan, insists, with his inimitable irreverence:

> Followers of the Way, simply follow your circumstances and fulfill your karma. When it's time to put on your robe, put it on; when you need to travel, walk onward; when you wish to sit down, just sit; and never have a single thought of entering Buddhahood.
>
> Followers of the Way, Buddhism requires no special efforts. You have only to lead your everyday life without seeking anything more—piss and shit, get dressed, eat your rice, and lie down when you are tired. (Addiss et al. 2008, 48)

Passages like these contain a rhetorical demonstration of freedom from formal rules and propriety, and these sometimes include even calling into question the need for formal meditation practice. To what extent this rhetoric actually influenced life on the ground for Chan/Zen practitioners is unclear. Certainly today, Zen monasteries are far from havens of spontaneous, free-form spirituality. Moreover, it would be mistaken to think of instructions like "do not think of good or evil; do not deal with right or wrong," or the admonition not to tamp down destructive emotional states and encourage felicitous ones as a complete break with the classical tradition of ethical cultivation. Tibetan meditation practices invariably begin with "preliminary practices" in which practitioners commit themselves to the basic moral principles of Buddhism, and ethical cultivation is also a given in Zen monastic contexts. Notwithstanding the tradition of "crazy wisdom" in Tibetan Buddhism and the literary depictions of Zen masters disregarding Buddhist ethics and teachings, the casting aside of ethical admonitions is usually seen as a temporary suspension for the purpose of a particular meditative practice, not a way to live one's entire life. There are famous exceptions: Zen masters who flagrantly broke monastic vows or Tantrikas who lived in cremation grounds flouting social conventions. But it seems that throughout much Buddhist history, whether one conceives of awakening as dependent on *creating* virtues and states of mind or as *uncovering* the awakened nature lying dormant within, what one actually does on the ground in pursuit of awakening is largely the same—meditate, study, and perform one's ethical and ritual duties.

Nevertheless, it is such rhetoric, rather than realities on the ground, that were influential in shaping contemporary attitudes toward meditation as something that goes beyond formal rules, institutional authority, and adherence to any particular system of thought or "religion." Romanticism and its countercultural descendants, with their valorization of rule-floating and expressive freedom, along with Humanistic psychology, with its affirmation of the inherent goodness of human beings, would be irresistibly drawn to the image of the Zen master as the epitome of individual insight, freedom, and creativity unencumbered by social norms and rules. This combines with a somewhat anti-intellectual strain of modern meditation that tends to devalue "thinking," concepts, and rational analysis as something that removes one from the immediate experience of real life. Innateist meditation is important to the genealogy of modern iterations of meditation in that it accounts for the idea, found in many recent articulations, that all one need do is calm the mind down, see the truth within and, from there, one will "naturally" do what is appropriate from one's essentially good innate nature. No need for complicated ethical training or development of particular characteristics and virtues. One has penetrated beyond external rules to the true source of morality within. Thus, the intellectual heritage of Romanticism, with its emphasis on interiority, self-expression, freedom from external rules, and deep feeling, was a magnet for innateist Buddhist thought and practice, particularly Zen (McMahan 2008, chapter 5).

Implications of Innateism, Insinuations of Emptiness

The deconstructive aspect of Buddhist meditation opens up a "depth" dimension to meditative practices. The delightfully loopy, paradoxical language surrounding it is designed to dismantle established patterns of thought, affect, and disposition, opening up a realm of the undefined, indeterminate, and unpredictable. Like the constructive aspects of meditation, it provides conceptual content—doctrines, philosophical positions, goals, values—but then disrupts one's appropriation of that content as settled truth, creating a kind of cognitive vacuum. It pushes language to its limits through dereification of fundamental structures of thought, particularly binary oppositions, giving way to the language of paradox. Such language at once provides ethical guidance and a philosophical outlook while denying them in any absolute sense, attempting to create a particular form of tranquil, attentive disequilibrium whose results might be unpredictable and structurally resistant to definitive analysis. This disequilibrium might serve to loosen up conceptual categories, encourage novelty, and alter the practitioner's sense of self and world. It is here where people report the feeling of being transported beyond ordinary thought, of all boundaries dissolving, of the ecstatic (or terrifying) feeling that things are not really how they seem in everyday life. This unsettling of the familiar topography of experience allows for envisioning alternative possibilities, configurations, and frameworks of interpretation. It has gone hand-in-hand with philosophical analysis as a method of critical interrogation of all assumptions and tacit beliefs.

And what of the relationship of this type of meditation to our theme of context and culture? While this dereification practice throws all categories, orientations, and dispositions into question, it does not simply reduce consciousness to a blank slate or make for utterly autonomous thought and action free from "external" influences. Virtually any meditation program, even the most minimalist, involves training of the mind and suggesting particular ways of thinking, feeling, acting, and valuing. These practices no doubt yield new insights, new self-knowledge, and even a new understanding of the world. And yet, like constructivist meditation, they too apply new lenses that reveal particularities that were obscured by the practitioner's default categories and intuitions, suggesting alternative values and opening up different ways of being in the world. This is why Ponlop Rinpoche, the contemporary teacher cited at the beginning of this chapter, insists that before one attempts nonconceptual Mahāmudrā meditation, one should have a clear understanding of the teachings surrounding the practice: "First, we learn with an open and interested mind what Mahamudra is. Then we reflect on and personalize that knowledge so that it becomes our own experience, rather than a theory. Then, having digested the meaning, we simply sit, going beyond knowing about Mahamudra to becoming one with it" (Ponlop 2020).

Although these meditative techniques are deconstructive, they inevitably involve reconstruction and imagination as well. Meditators who seek to discover the truth of emptiness and interdependence have expectations of how their lives will be transformed by this realization, even if they manage to avoid projecting such expectations during the actual practice. Books, talks, and tradition guide the practitioner's intuitions. One is trained to "see" emptiness, to experience the world as interdependent, or perhaps to imagine the universe as a conscious, expansive process of infinite activity. One is guided to look for hints of emptiness, interdependence, or buddha-nature in one's day-to-day life, to notice connection rather than disconnection, to configure one's relationships with others in particular ways—as interdependent processes in a common matrix, like eddies in a stream, rather than as independent entities bumping into each other like billiard balls. Such meditations, and the culture surrounding them, encourage the enacting of particular habits of perception, the training of the imagination, an attunement to certain features of the world rather than others, and a disciplining of one's interpretations.

The deconstructive features of these practices are always, therefore, in a dialectical relationship with constructive, interpretive elements, conceptual frameworks, strategies of interpretation, and imaginings. Theravāda Buddhists will be trained to analyze their experience as having no permanent self. Those committed to the buddha-nature doctrine will search their minds for their innate buddhahood. Hindus will be trained to search their minds for the supreme, undying Self. No matter what that final reality is (or if such a reality is itself a myth), the process of getting there is one of shaping the mind and body to experience things and imagine one's overall situation in certain ways; of crafting a new phenomenological reality. Imagining what it is like to be enlightened, analyzing complex teachings and doctrines, imitating the behavior of enlightened ones, performing calmness in social situations is inevitably a part of the process.

We can see how this works in some of the meditation instructions in the Chan/Zen tradition. On the one hand, they can be relentlessly dereifying and deconstructive, calling into question every moment of the meditator's experience, suggesting that it is an illusion—the fostering of what the tradition calls "great doubt." Yet, on the other hand, they also insist that every element of the illusion is itself the very nature of reality, the very mind of the Buddha, the cosmic mind. One is asked to step back from everything one encounters—material objects, other people, dogs and cats, stalks of bamboo—and insist to oneself that the way one is apprehending and conceiving them is flawed and distorted, like mistaking the reflection of the moon in the water for the moon itself. Withdraw all attachment and personal associations with the things and one will see them as they are—manifestations of the one true Reality. The tension between construction and deconstruction lies in the fact that, upon hearing such teachings one cannot help but imagine what it might be like to apprehend things in this way. One is, in fact, being asked to imagine a very different world, one in which all plurality is contained within an overarching unity. Part of the unique effort of Zen and other innateist forms of meditation is to balance the feat of cutting off all imaginings while imagining (perhaps while trying not to imagine) what it is that one is aiming for, what it is to see—to *be*—the world as buddha-nature. One must, through imagination, infuse transcendence into immanence, and strain the interpretive capacities to see the flower, the pebble, the act of eating or defecation as sacred.

Thus practitioners are trained, not just through formal meditation itself, but through literature, dharma talks, and the surrounding culture, to create a new imaginary; to suspect that the ordinary leaf, stone, or bowl, is something mysterious and profound, harboring the full luminosity of the cosmos. One learns to entertain the apparently absurd proposition that despite the appearance of old age, sickness, death, war, and chaos, the world—*this* world—is perfection, a pristine manifestation of buddha-nature. To learn to experience things in such a way requires effort, for it goes against the compelling and competing vision of ordinariness—the tree is just a tree, the bowl just a bowl, death just death. To pull it off, one must rely on something that is often downplayed in modern accounts of Buddhism: *śraddhā*—faith. The Zen tradition frames this as a tension, necessary for producing the effort for practice, between great faith and great doubt.

Modern people might well experience such a tension acutely—and somewhat differently—than the ancients, for we live, according to some accounts, in a disenchanted world, bereft of the gods, spirits, or a hidden, divine order. Actually, such disenchantment is likely not as universal as its theorists have suspected, but no matter; it is an ailment at least of the educated class that brought Buddhism into the frameworks of modernity. And part of what created an opportunity for Zen to flourish in its modern iterations was the lingering hope among the globalizers of Zen that the despirited world brought by science and secularism still veiled a sacred order—that the tree and the bowl, with their spiritless chemical reactions and mechanical atomic rotations, were themselves enlivened by this hidden order. In the modern world, this combination of dereification and resacralization allowed the new imaginary of the secular to fuse with the imagery of the Buddhist sacred.

A final aspect to the tension between the constructive and deconstructive aspects of meditation that has had a significant impact on the contemporary practice of meditation is between the "single-practice" model and a more multiform model. Japanese Buddhist traditions have often espoused the ideal of the single, essential practice that permeates one's life. In Nichiren traditions, it's chanting the homage to the *Lotus Sūtra: nam myōho renge kyō*. In Zen, it is seated meditation—*shikantaza*, "just sitting," or "single-minded sitting." The idea is not that one just sits all of one's life but that there is a quality of mind with "one taste" to be cultivated in seated meditation and that this quality is to be carried forth into all activities. This streamlined approach will allow one to encounter all of life's circumstances with focus and directness, and to spontaneously respond appropriately and skillfully. Some

Theravāda-derived Vipassanā traditions adopted this attitude as well, emphasizing a single, specific method of meditation and minimizing much of the philosophical, ethical, and ritual elements that traditionally surrounded the practice. This approach gets absorbed into much contemporary literature on mindfulness, which also suggests that having the quality of mindfulness in all circumstances will facilitate the successful navigation of life in its variegated facets. Mindfulness will make for better family relations, health, work performance, sex, pain management, eating, and, well, virtually everything. This, in turn, has led to a common complaint that mindfulness is being presented as a panacea that mitigates all problems and enhances all good things.

To illustrate how this "single-practice" approach contrasts with a more constructivist, virtue-building approach, it is worth quoting at length the American Theravāda monk, Thanissaro Bhikkhu, who offers a critique of contemporary Vipassanā, along with an interesting bit of historical interpretation:

> The idea of creating meditation retreats came basically in the late 19th or early 20th century, the same time when the assembly line was invented, breaking jobs down into little tiny parts that you do repetitively. This approach to physical work was efficient and effective, so it became the model for a lot of meditation retreats and for the methods taught on those retreats. You take one method and you just apply it again and again and again. But a lot gets left out in that approach. It's like exercising only one muscle in your body, so that the muscle gets strengthened all out of proportion to the rest of your body. And that can't be healthy.
>
> It's better to think of meditation as a training for the whole mind, as exercise for the whole mind. You have to train the whole mind in all the virtues of maturity and heedfulness. In other words, you need to develop the ability to anticipate dangers, particularly dangers in your own behavior, and to figure out what you can do to prevent them. (Thānissaro 2008)

Thanissaro's position highlights the potential problems with a too-streamlined approach and recalls Evan Thompson's insistence that mindfulness is "a host of cognitive, affective, and bodily skills in situated action" (Thompson 2017, 52). This is not really a Zen-versus-Theravāda issue but one that cuts across various Buddhist meditation traditions. Again, on the ground, Zen monks in training monasteries are cultivating virtues and developing diverse skills, despite the "one-practice" rhetoric in the literature. But, as is often the case, when tracing the influences of Buddhist traditions on contemporary mindfulness practices, we often find these influences in selected bits and pieces of literature rather than practice on the ground. These bits and pieces highlight ideas and attitudes that can speak to contemporary issues and that can take up residence in particular spaces in the architecture of modern secularism. In the following chapters we attempt to map out some of that architecture and show how certain Buddhist themes and practices have come to occupy these spaces.

Let's recapitulate the argument so far, before moving to another phase of the book. Of the great myriad of Buddhist meditative practices, various cultural filters have kept most of them from taking root in the modern West, while certain cultural magnets have drawn forth, and transformed, a small number. These have coalesced into a Standard Version of mindfulness meditation, which has been stripped of most Buddhist language so that it can occupy secular spaces. It has been studied extensively by scientists and, therefore, gained considerable legitimacy and cultural capital. This, in turn, has allowed it to quickly become a widely used therapeutic tool for treatment of countless ailments, as well as a technique for living well more generally.

I have questioned an interpretation, popular among some practitioners and scientific researchers, of how such practices work; that is, that they allow practitioners to obtain a clear, neutral view of "objective" truths in the mind, truths that transcend cultural context and personal perspective, be they the stream of consciousness or "laws of nature" manifest internally. I have also suggested that much of the scientific research involving brain imaging, and especially the promise of mapping states of meditative consciousness (or even enlightenment itself) through technological measurement, is less promising than many hope and that they rest on problematic models of the mind.

Instead, I have offered a more constructivist approach to the work that meditation does, one that emphasizes the way these practices are embedded in social imaginaries and draw from a repertoire of concepts, affective dispositions, and ethical orientations in particular cultural contexts and traditions. As the SP shows, Pali meditative practices not only engage the attention but also engage the intellect and emotions, encouraging certain states of mind and discouraging others, fostering certain intellectual understandings and urging practitioners to dwell within particular portraits of self and world. In this sense, they are practices of self-transformation that aim at creating certain kinds of subjects, crafting character and honing particular skills and ways of being in the world. Part of the way they do this is that they also contain, in tension with the constructive aspects, deconstructive aspects that call into question and, in some cases, disrupt and dismantle habitual ways of being. Thus, the constructive and deconstructive exist in a kind of creative tension that fosters transformative potentials. Practices that emphasize the deconstructive side can seem antinomian and often call for cutting off conceptualization, reducing all appearances and goals for self-cultivation to illusion. Yet they, too, implicitly foster certain ways of being in the world within particular traditions, whether those traditions are orthodox versions of Buddhism or contemporary North American secularism.

This picture leaves some questions unaddressed. If meditation is not simply a method for coming to objective internal truths, how do we conceive of insights that practitioners claim to have? Also, if it is not a means to a kind of transcultural freedom that allows one to extract the mind from external influence and cultural conditioning and unleashing a purely self-generated autonomy, is there another way to conceive of their emancipatory potentials? Do people, in other words, really acquire a sense of enhanced freedom through them, and in what sense—or are they just trading one set of cultural constraints for another? While thinking through these questions, we will also consider a few examples of how the practices have become infused into various de facto ideals present in modern (and late-modern) contexts that are distinct from those in some of the more "traditional" ones in which they arose. This will allow us to see with more specificity what it might mean to say that they have been "modernized" or "secularized," and to make more sense of the sometimes-novel purposes to which they are put.

PART III
MEDITATION AND THE ETHICAL SUBJECT

8

Secularism and the Ethic of Appreciation

Dispatches from the Worlds of Meditation: 8a
Take a moment to take in the surrounding environment, focusing on what you see around you. Notice whether it is quiet or busy. As you continue walking, direct your attention to the sounds, then the sensations in the air. How does it feel against your skin? As you continue on the walk, settle into this rhythm. This exercise will help you focus on the present, and notice and appreciate the little things we generally take for granted.
— **From the website of Headspace, a meditation app[1]**

Dispatches from the Worlds of Meditation: 8b
"I sat and sat and sat. I meditated *hard*, over a long period of time. And I was still a shit."
— **Buddhist Studies scholar and former practitioner, in conversation with author and a Zen teacher, 2013.**

The Subject of Ethics and the Ethical Subject

I've argued that at least part of "work" that meditative practices do is that they create and foster specific modes of being in the world within particular social, historical, and political contexts and that these are always tied to a moral or ethical vision of how one *should* be in the world. We have seen that, in their foundational phases, Buddhist meditative practices embodied a tension between distant, transcendent goals (awakening, nirvana) and proximate goals involving how to live in this world. Throughout much of the history of Buddhism, practitioners of meditation were mostly monastics, therefore the ethics attached to meditation were the ethics of monastic life. And yet, these practices have changed, developed, and expanded over many centuries, adapting to diverse cultural and political contexts and contributing

Rethinking Meditation. David L. McMahan, Oxford University Press. © Oxford University Press 2023.
DOI: 10.1093/oso/9780197661741.003.0008

to different projects and moral visions. The ethics attached to meditative practices have changed and multiplied over time, and today they are undergoing unprecedented transformations as they seep into multifarious domains of life previously foreign to them.

The way the relationship between meditation and ethics is often conceived in modern Buddhist and Buddhist-influenced literature is that meditation brings one to moral clarity from an authoritative source within. Meditation might be conceived, for example, as the empirical observation of the workings of the mind, including the universal causes of mental suffering, and this observation allows one to choose courses of thought, feeling, and action that will not bring about further suffering. Or it might be conceived as a means of tapping into a wellspring of natural goodness, clearing away distractions and social conditioning to arrive at a hidden reservoir of authentic virtue.

The relationship between meditation and ethics becomes murkier, however, when considering the intricacies of everyday ethical deliberation in a particular socio-political context. Consider the following examples: an American meditator comes to the realization that the causes of suffering are not just internal and individual but also systemic; therefore, she resolves to work diligently, not only to root out racial prejudice in herself but also to join a local Black Lives Matter group dedicated to combating the often-harsh treatment of Black Americans at the hands of law enforcement. Another individual, a Burmese monk, sits mindfully in his monastery and comes to the conviction that the *sāsana*, the Buddha's teachings and practices, is threatened in Myanmar by the Muslim population. According to a revered monk he has recently heard preaching, they will turn Myanmar into a Muslim country if they are not stopped. Out of compassion for his fellow Buddhists and devotion to his Buddhist homeland and its Burmese race, he resolves to join the Organization for the Protection of Race and Religion (known by the acronym Ma Ba Tha), which propagates anti-Muslim rhetoric and has provided the rationale for the brutal ethnic cleansing of the Rohingya from Myanmar. The Buddha's teachings cannot continue their benevolent mission, he reasons, if it is extinguished by outsiders.

Both of these individuals are deploying Buddhist meditative techniques for discerning moral truths. Clearly, however, they have different underlying ethical frameworks that their meditative practices help them clarify, magnify, and act on. We need not understate the horror of Buddhist-supported genocide to notice that the monk's views are, nevertheless, constructed from parts of Buddhism combined—if perversely—with the social imaginary of his time and place. Both meditators' ethical conclusions come about through a complicated negotiation between history, tradition, and present opinion among their peers and various media. This negotiation involves the continuance of ethical argument within a tradition that is inevitably meeting unprecedented circumstances, drawing upon repertoires of available concepts, ideals, and narratives, as well as creatively innovating by the selective reinterpretation of tradition and novel application of its principles. That different meditators could come to such radically different ethical stances calls into question the claim that meditation brings about universal ethical insights or that accomplished meditators inevitably come to the same moral vision.

Even moral concepts that might seem unambiguous, like loving-kindness or compassion, inevitably take on particular significance in specific social imaginaries. Thus skill in killing human beings who are threatening one's family, community, nation, emperor, and the Dharma itself can and has been presented as selfless, compassionate action (Victoria 2006; Jerryson and Juergensmeyer 2010). The ethical insights that meditation confers may provide new understanding and exceed the boundaries of one's normative ethical context, but they are always nevertheless embedded in that context—the ideas, ideals, convictions, outrages, and the incessant impingement of events unfolding in the present—and must be made relevant to it. The moral imperatives that meditators discover in states of deep concentration cannot be removed altogether from the dominant conceptions of morality that they have read about or heard from their neighbors, nor from the rough and tumble of normal ethical deliberation. Moreover, meditation in and of itself seems to guarantee no particular fidelity to ethical principles; that is, it doesn't automatically make you a better person, as demonstrated most recently by the many cases of sexual abuse by accomplished meditation masters in American Buddhist centers in recent decades (Gleig 2019). Evidently, you can meditate for over 10,000 hours and still be a jerk.[2]

In the next four chapters, I aim to map out some contours of the relationship between (relatively) secularized Buddhist and Buddhist-derived meditation and several secular ethical ideals. I am not focusing primarily on particular ethical injunctions—whether one should consume alcohol, have sex outside of marriage, or fight in a war. Rather, I want to provide a sketch of certain components of the substructure of modern secularism—the often-implicit network of values operative in contemporary liberal societies—and to show how Buddhist meditation has come to inhabit this substructure. By secularized meditative practices, I do not mean practices occurring exclusively outside the institutional spheres of Buddhism, nor only mindfulness practices that have been stripped clean of Buddhist terminology. Rather, I mean styles of meditative practice that have emerged through the intertwining of complex, multifaceted traditions of Buddhism and the ideological infrastructure of secularity and liberalism. I hope to show how this infrastructure often provides the implicit "why" and "how" of meditation today.

Before elucidating the particular facets of this infrastructure, however, I want to address some further points about the relationship between Buddhism and secularism.

Secularism and the Secular Meditator

The imperative in much contemporary meditation for avoiding the supernatural and focusing on interiority and this-worldly concerns is itself conditioned by what we might think of as the dominant discourse of the late modern liberal societies: secularism. We cannot address the Standard Version of meditation without understanding that it has been configured specifically within the parameters of the secular. For the past 150 years or so, Buddhists and Buddhist enthusiasts have often presented the Dharma to the world more as a philosophy or "way of life" than a religion. Revitalization movements of the colonial period de-emphasized the ritual, devotional, and supernatural elements of Buddhism ubiquitous in Asia and highlighted its philosophical, ethical, and psychological features, tailoring these in dialogue with various strands of secular (and its new cousin, "spiritual," McMahan 2012) thought in the West—psychology, transcendentalism, rationalism, romanticism, and liberalism. This endeavor was spearheaded mostly by Asian Buddhists keen to rethink Buddhism in light of emerging global currents of thought; it was also a strategic effort to rebuff the denigrating images of Buddhism and the subjugation of Buddhist populations under colonialism. These reformers translated Buddhism into the philosophical and religious terms of the European colonial powers in order, in turn, to critique those powers and stake an intellectual, ethical, and cultural claim for Buddhism in the world of globalizing modernity. Thus, Buddhism in the nineteenth century began to be framed as a psychology, a system of rational ethics, and a source of spiritual wisdom for an increasingly mechanized, industrialized, and dispirited world. And, indeed, Buddhism has gained a great deal of prestige by being cast as a kind of secular spirituality that mitigates the dehumanizing forces of industrial and postindustrial modernity but does not transgress the dominant discourse of the scientific worldview and the liberal political order.

When people today think of the increasing effects of secularism on Buddhist meditation, they might ask questions like: *should* meditation be secularized? Is secularized meditation authentic? Does it strip away too many essential elements of Buddhism? Rather than weigh in on the merits and defects of a secularized meditation, I want to think through some issues involving how two long, variegated traditions—Buddhist meditation and modern secularism—converge. Often when people speak to the issue of secularized meditation, they speak in terms of explicit beliefs. Might meditation mitigate the possibility of rebirth as a hungry ghost or in a hell realm? Does it foster supernormal powers like telepathy or teleportation? Might it be helpful in warding off evil spirits? The fewer things like these that meditators believe, the more secular their practice, some would say. These kinds of questions play an important role in secularizing meditation, especially because one common use of the term *secularism* today involves explicit beliefs. In fact, there is a Secular Buddhism movement today that explicitly rejects elements of Buddhism like rebirth, traditional cosmology, supernatural beings, and others that do not conform to modern scientific understanding of the world and the human being.[3] But we might also consider the ways in which what we might call *secularity*—the pervasive, naturalistic zeitgeist of the times, the dominant discourse of modernity, the implicit ideology of public discourse—structures not just explicit beliefs but also more subtle ways of being in the world, experiencing oneself, and navigating one's life possibilities. Secularity in this sense functions as a kind of background ideology that is so pervasive it often goes unnoticed. It is tied inevitably to secularism as a political project (the separation of church and state), but also to particular conceptions and configurations of the self (an independent, subjective mind confronting an objective world of facts), and, indeed, particular notions of what is religious and what is secular (religion as having to do primarily with beliefs, internal experience, emotions, and the secular having to do with rationality, public discourse, and politics).

The binary of religious and secular does not refer to some objective state of things in the world but is a historically particular way of dividing things up, of constituting human subjects, and of framing institutions like public schools, churches, governmental organizations, and the courts. As a sociopolitical project, secularism itself is rooted in an attempt to cleave rational deliberation in the public square from "religion," which is conceived as a matter of private, individual belief. In ways that Buddhists should understand, the religious and the secular are not mere facts in the world, but, like many (all?) binary oppositions, they are coconstituted, intertwined, and culturally and historically contingent. The religious and the secular, in other words, are interdependently arisen, recently invented ways of configuring the world and constituting our experience.[4] Nevertheless, if secularism is, in fact, the dominant discourse of much of the developed world, it has already deeply structured the way many Buddhists practice their tradition. Because Buddhism made headway in Europe and North America—and was revitalized in Asia—in large part by being framed as aligned with a secular, scientific orientation and distancing itself from things that were typically associated with "religion" and, especially, "superstition," much Buddhist meditation today, whether in the monastery or the health club, is already secularized to some extent.

This does not mean that secularized meditation has been stripped of all "religious" purposes and concepts. Again, when I refer to "secularized meditation," I am not simply referring to meditation that occurs outside of religious institutions in the YMCA or the conference room of tech companies. It is, instead, meditation that has taken on the rhetorical and conceptual apparatus of secularism, rationalism, science, and liberalism. This does not necessarily mean that people practicing relatively secularized meditation never believe in spirits, rebirth, or magical powers—or that they don't think of what they are doing as "spiritual" in the contemporary sense of the word. It refers, rather, to meditation whose object is not defined solely in the categories of a religious tradition—nirvana, awakening, spiritual insight, magical powers—but in terms of secular categories—laws of nature, the unconscious mind, the cultivation of certain brain states. Today, even Buddhist monks will often describe meditation in these terms.

This structuring of meditation as a secular/spiritual, rather than "religious," endeavor has had specific, concrete effects on the shape of contemporary mindfulness and meditative practices. The Standard Version of mindfulness practiced in North America and Europe—and increasingly around the globe—has been configured explicitly to the contours of secularism in the United States.[5] Mindfulness-based stress reduction (MBSR), which has become immensely popular among clinicians, educators, and corporations, is an avowedly "secular" mindfulness program developed by Jon Kabat-Zinn and derived from a combination of Vipassana, or Insight Meditation, and Zen Buddhist forms of meditation. Buddhist language, however, was carefully excised from the program so that it could be taught in American public institutions that are categorized as secular. The secularization of meditation is not just a matter of style, however, but also of law. In the United States, it is illegal to promote a particular religious view in public institutions. In Kabat-Zinn's program, the practices were simplified and reformulated in the language of medicine and psychology, braided into strands of the United States' particular version of secularism, its legal specificities, and its criteria for legitimacy and prestige.[6] This reformulation, however, was only one of the more recent moves in a long process of the secularization of Buddhist meditation that extends back to the nineteenth century. Within this short period of time, the institutional home of this kind of practice has shifted from being nearly exclusively in Buddhist monasteries to some of the most prominent and powerful secular institutions in the world: Goldman-Sachs, Harvard Medical School,

Google, the US military, the British National Health Service. It would be naive to think these Buddhist-derived practices that now reside in such new institutional environments are not radically repurposed as techniques for fostering the skills and sensibilities sanctioned by such institutions. This is why this is clearly such an unprecedented moment in the long, winding history of these practices, when they now mutate into countless subspecies commandeered for multifarious purposes.

And yet, perhaps not so multifarious, for most are enfolded within the implicit background of secularity, which structures and delimits their shape. It is difficult to see this, because secularism has become the publicly sanctioned way of seeing things, the default common-sense that constitutes not just rational beliefs about, say, what causes things to happen (illness is caused by a virus, not a malign spirit) but also vague intuitions and sensibilities that might not rise to explicit conceptualization. Secularity in this vaguer sense is less visible, but nonetheless shapes one's sense of life and one's available choices, structuring one's habitual intuitions.[7] That secularity has this dominant place does not mean that everyone has "secular beliefs." Many, of course, still believe in supernatural beings, heavens and hells, and astrology. But the status of secularism, with its epistemological wing, the sciences, as the officially sanctioned public discourse, the discourse of the public educational system and of political deliberation, makes it mandatory for a novel practice or idea to negotiate with secular normativity. Contemporary Buddhist and Buddhist-derived meditation practices have been molded significantly by this negotiation.

The secularization of meditation is not simply a matter of extracting the supposedly pure practice from the packaging of religious language, symbols, and cosmology in which it has been immersed, like removing a crystal wrapped in tissue paper from its box. In his analysis of secularism, Charles Taylor cautions against seeing the emergence of secularism as a "subtraction story," that is, the gradual subtraction of something called "religion" from something (there all along) called the "secular" (Taylor 2007). Scholars of the secular are quite skeptical today of the narrative of global secularization popular in the twentieth century, in which, in the face of science, technology, and capitalism, the world uniformly becomes less and less religious—or religion becomes a merely private matter, largely irrelevant to social and political life. Instead, many have emphasized that secularism is coconstituted with religion, and in ways deeply implicated in the relations between "the West" and Asia. The secularism paradigm is rooted in the European Enlightenment, with its valorization of reason, choice, activity, personal autonomy, and individualism, not to mention its historical framing of these virtues as the properties of "the West," while "the East" was often associated with the irrational, the mysterious, the feminine, the passive, and the collective (King 1999). Peter van der Veer points out that "the very distinction between religious and secular is a product of the Enlightenment that was used in Orientalism to draw a sharp opposition between irrational, religious behavior of the Oriental and rational secularism, which enabled the westerner to rule the Oriental" (Breckenridge and van der Veer 1993, 39). Talal Asad similarly emphasizes how the binaries of East and West were mapped onto other binaries, such as reason and emotion, knowledge and belief, natural and supernatural, sacred and profane (Asad 2003). And the secular side of these binaries has wielded real-world power, in the hands of the state, not just to delineate and classify religion but to manage it. There is also a compelling case to be made that secularism, particularly in its American incarnation, is heavily inflected toward the racial category of "white," as well as male and "civilized" (Kahn and Lloyd 2016). Indeed, part of what has been filtered in the process of secularizing Buddhism in the West has often been elements of Buddhism that were specifically marked as "Asian," and therefore threatening to the dominant racial and power hierarchies, in favor of purportedly culturally neutral mindfulness practices that were scientifically legitimated and stripped of all "cultural baggage" (Hsu 2021). Of course, the apparatus of secularism is just as much a matter of "cultural baggage" as incense and prostration before statues of the Buddha.

Part of the revitalization of Buddhism during the colonial period involved attempting to reverse the value of some of these binaries: Buddhist apologists presented Asia generally, and Buddhism in particular, as bringing ancient wisdom, spirituality, and humaneness to a world remade by the West's skewed emphasis on rationality, technological achievement, industry, economic vitality, and military conquest. And yet, these reformers nonetheless adopted secular language to describe what meditation does and how it works: that is, it clears away obscuring emotions and thoughts, irrational personal reactions to circumstances, false beliefs, and the like, to reveal the "real," objective facts underneath. In this sense, contemporary reformulations of meditation have often adopted the logic of secularism and science, presenting it as the search for an objective truth free of social, cultural, and emotional obscuration. That truth has been construed to parallel scientific truth in that it isolates knowledge from belief, fact from value judgment, the concrete real of "experience" from the fictional story of the "ego," the inner data of contemplative science from the irrational speculations and passions of "religion" or "superstition."

Buddhist and Buddhist-derived meditative practices, therefore, have become intertwined with the social imaginary of secularism and liberalism, adopting a this-worldly bearing and taking on board the values prevalent in liberal democracies. Below, I inquire into some particular ways that these practices have come to be means of realizing a few of these values—values that are deeply embedded in the contemporary ethos and that, nevertheless, sometimes pick up resonant Buddhist values and, in other instances, run against their grain.

The Underlying Ideals of Secular Meditation

What should meditation do? Of what values should it be put in service? What kind of emotional dispositions, intellectual capacities, and aesthetic sensibilities should it help cultivate? What good might it do for individuals and societies? What kind of knowledge can one glean from it? What kind of freedom might it confer? When people ask such questions today, the answers do not come from the Buddhist traditions alone but from a complex interweaving of discursive threads from multiple cultural histories that entwine in the pervasive atmosphere of late-modern secularity. Below I sketch several components of what I think of as the ethical infrastructure of modern secular ethics into which Buddhist meditation has been absorbed and to which it has made distinct contributions. They are:

- the ethic of appreciation
- the ethic of authenticity
- the ethic of autonomy
- the ethic of interdependence

Each of these has its own history and its own ideals, which have magnetically drawn Buddhist meditative practices to them according to their particular ethical logics. These different "ethics" do not all fit together to make a consistent whole but, in fact, reveal the tensions between various opposing tendencies endemic to the current age, particularly the tension between meditation as a private exploration of the individual's interior—or a facilitator of individual interior freedom—and the inevitable embeddedness of any meditator in a social, cultural, and political context. The first three ethics—those of appreciation, authenticity, and autonomy—lean toward an individualistic interpretation of meditation, while the ethic of interdependence has emerged more recently as a counterbalance emphasizing the permeability of individuals, their openness to the world, to others, and to the cosmos.

"Appreciate Your Life": Strawberries and the Ethic of Appreciation

A man traveling across a field encountered a tiger. He fled, the tiger after him. Coming to a precipice, he caught hold of the root of a wild vine and swung himself down over the edge. The tiger sniffed at him from above. Trembling, the man looked down to where, far below, another tiger was waiting to eat him. Only the vine sustained him. Two mice one white and one black, little by little started to gnaw away the vine. The man saw a luscious strawberry near him. Grasping the vine with one hand, he plucked the strawberry with the other. How sweet it tasted!

This well-known story is from one of the first widely read works on Zen published in English, *Zen Flesh, Zen Bones*, compiled and published by Paul Reps in 1957. It incorporates stories from several sources, including a book published in 1919 called *101 Zen Stories* (Senzaki 1919), which in turn drew mostly from a thirteenth-century Japanese collection, the *Shasekishū*, and a kōan collection, *The Gateless Gate* (Jpn: *Mumonkan*).

Ask anyone today the meaning of the story and they will likely give the same answer: *carpe diem*; Seize the day! Enjoy life while it lasts; live life to the fullest; savor the simple pleasures of life while you can; or, in the words of the title of a book by a Japanese Zen teacher who taught for much of his life in Los Angeles: *Appreciate Your Life* (Maezumi 2002). Many philosophers and religious thinkers have emphasized that profound awareness of one's mortality—being toward death, in Heidegger's words—changes the way one lives and feels life. Anyone who has had a serious illness or accident knows something about this. You don't take your life for granted anymore. So this story presents an illustration of being able to appreciate the sweetness of whatever the moment brings in the face of the situation we are all inevitably in—hanging on for life while the white and black mice of passing days and nights nibble away at our remaining time. The "Zen attitude," the story suggests, is to fully appreciate and savor each moment in unblinking awareness of our precarious circumstance. Meditation, we might further infer, fosters this appreciation.

There exist, however, other iterations of the story that imply an altogether different message, including versions in ancient Buddhist and Hindu texts. The Buddhist one is in the *Lalitavistara*, a fourth-century Sanskrit account of the life of the Buddha, from which it was incorporated into a Chinese sūtra (Taisho 217). In this text, the man is chased by an elephant instead of a tiger, he falls into a well instead of off a cliff, and two rats, rather than mice, nibble the vine. Below him is a great serpent, and four snakes come from the sides of the well attempting to bite him. Instead of the strawberry, there is a beehive from which drops of honey fall into his mouth while bees swarm and sting him. And brushfires burn the tree branch to which he clings. The Buddha, who is relating this story, details what the various elements represent (for example, the elephant is impermanence, the fire is old age, the serpent below, death). The five drops of honey represent the five desires: for food and drink, sleep, sex, wealth, and fame. He leaves no ambiguity about the moral of the story: "That is why, great king, you should know that birth, old age, illness, and death are quite terrible. You should always remember them, and not become a slave to your desires."[8] In a version found in the Hindu epic, the *Mahābhārata*, the story is put into the mouth of a Jain monk, who explains that the drops of honey are trivial pleasures that people become attached to and consume insatiably, distracting them from the spiritual life. He mocks the doomed man for craving the superficial pleasure of the honey in the face of his precarious situation (Embree 1988 [1958], 59–61).

The story of how this tale migrates from the world-weary ethos of ancient ascetic communities in India to the back pockets of world-affirming, strawberry-eating seekers in the 1960s is long, complicated, and fascinating. I'll only mention a few of the stops.[9] The story of the Buddha's life told in the *Lalitavistara*, containing within it our story of the unfortunate falling man, was picked up by the Manicheans and transformed into the tale of Barlaam and Josaphat (the latter's name is likely derived from the term "bodhisattva"). An Arabic version circulated in eighth-century Persia, and from there it was adapted to Christianity and attributed to St. John Chrysorrhoas of Damascus (675–749). In this version the man is transfixed with tasting the honey and, failing to notice a ladder his friend extends to him, falls and is devoured by the dragon below, now representing Satan.

The story of Barlaam and Josaphat circulated throughout Europe and the Middle East for centuries and was translated into dozens of languages. In the nineteenth century, Leo Tolstoy used the story of the man in the well as the centerpiece of his autobiographical work, *A Confession*, where he saw it as an expression of the futility of his life up to the point of his radical personal transformation and embracing of a liberal, pacifist understanding of the teachings of Jesus. Tolstoy's autobiography, in turn, had a profound influence on a young Indian lawyer in the late nineteenth century—Mohandās Gandhi—who would incorporate it into his own revolutionary teachings. So the story made its way back to India after becoming a part of most of the major religious traditions of the world and attaining new meanings and significance in each one. Meanwhile, around the same time Gandhi encountered it, a Zen monk named Nyogen Senzaki (1876–1958), one of the first Zen monks to teach in the United States, compiled and helped translate a version of the story of the man in the well—which had all the while been circulating in Asia, both independently and as a part of the *Lalitavistara* and other texts—into the version we have now in English in the book *101 Zen Stories*, which became a part of Reps's slim, pocket-sized volume, which is still in print and part of essential Zen reading in America. It is not altogether clear to me how the various changes from the *Lalitavistara* version to Senzaki's version came to be over the centuries, nor how the moral of the story transformed from "Your days are numbered; renounce trivial sense pleasures and pursue awakening" to "Appreciate your life, seize the day, relish the strawberry." Whether Senzaki himself made this change or it picked up more world-affirming tones in its migration through Chinese and Japanese cultures, he must have known that the *carpe diem* version would resonate with the optimistic, world-embracing ethos of English-speaking world in the early twentieth century.

The journey of this story illustrates how texts, works of art, poems, rituals are never fixed in their meaning. They yield up new interpretations in new contexts, as novel meanings are coaxed out of them by new social imaginaries, and people tweak them to resonate with prevailing ideals and assumptions. All of this is a rather roundabout way of illustrating that the ethic of renunciation so pervasive in early Buddhist literature often fades into invisibility in modernized Buddhisms and is largely displaced by what I am calling the ethic of appreciation. This ethic entails an affirmation of the implicit value of the physical world, the senses, and the ordinary experience of ordinary people.

The ethic of appreciation contrasts strikingly with the ethic of world-renunciation that dominates the early Buddhist literature. This literature contains not only a systematic worldview—an account of how the world is—it contains detailed training in how to *feel* toward it. It is part of a broader Indian ascetic literature that, as we have discussed in chapters 4 and 5, attempts to train the mind to see things in particular ways, develop particular virtues, sensibilities, aesthetic responses, and affective habits. According to the suttas and the Vinaya, monastics must train themselves in detachment from the world. They are to cultivate indifference, for example, to the eight worldly concerns: hope for gain and fear of loss; hope for fame and fear of disgrace; hope for praise and fear of blame; hope for pleasure and fear of pain (AN 8.5). They are to see the world as something that cannot possibly bring about satisfaction, as something fleeting and unreliable, deceptive and beguiling. They should become disenchanted with it and withdraw emotional investment in seeking satisfaction from it. They are to imagine the interior of bodies to counter attraction to physical beauty, cultivate revulsion at physiological processes like digestion and sex, and take opportunities to view corpses to ameliorate illusions of permanence and vivify the inevitability of death. They are to shun attachment to family and avoid seeking solace in the inevitably fragile and unstable human relationships. The world—"all of this"—is to be seen as a "mass of suffering."

There is another side to this, however. These attitudes exist in counterpoint to advice in the suttas on good family relations and the need to cultivate particular social emotions like love, compassion, and taking joy in others' happiness. In later literature, readers are advised to cultivate the kind of love toward all living beings that a mother has for her only son. The Buddha gives advice to kings on worldly affairs and is clearly invested in the well-being of people, animals, and society. So on the textual level, a tension exists between an ethic of detachment and disengagement and a more this-worldly ethic of compassion and engagement. We should also keep in mind that these textual admonitions are expressions of ideals that don't necessarily reflect realities on the ground. Gregory Schopen's research, for example, shows that canonical prescriptive texts are not a reliable guide for judging how monastics actually lived and practiced (2004). Also, we should remember the wide array of this-worldly practices Buddhists have developed that were oriented toward physical health, worldly prosperity, and a fortunate rebirth this side of nirvana. We must, therefore, be careful not to overstate the otherworldliness of early Buddhism or suggest that it has an unrelentingly negative view on embodied life. Yet in this early literature, there is undeniably a steady leitmotif of antipathy toward the processes of biological life, an emphasis on the fleetingness of things in the flow of *saṃsāra*, and the ultimate futility of finding satisfaction within the material world of change. A great deal of Buddhist literature attempts to navigate this tension between the ascetic ethic of renunciation and transcendence—which calls for detachment from the phenomenal world—and an ethic of compassion, which calls for deep empathetic engagement with living beings. A prominent position in Mahāyāna literature, for example, is to lean more toward amplifying the ethic of compassion to the point that the ultimate goal of *parinirvāṇa* (nirvana after death) is mitigated by the bodhisattva vow not to leave the world behind until all living beings have achieved awakening.

The message of the early version of the story of the man in the well—as well as the corpse meditations and contemplations of the repugnance of the body—is not that one should appreciate one's life, with its delicious honey drops, beautiful scenery, exquisite scents and tastes, and other physical delights. It is, rather, that such sensual engagement merely entraps one further in the cycle of *saṃsāra*. Granted, Buddhist traditions are not univocal in this, and we shouldn't suppose that all appreciation of ordinary life and physical beauty were somehow foreign to Buddhists. Tantric literature sometimes reverses the devaluation of the physical, valorizing the body and physiological processes, seeing them as essential to liberation:

> So one should not torment oneself with austerities,
> Abandoning the five sense-objects.
> One should notice beauty as it comes along,
> And listen to the sound.
>
> One should smell the odor
> And savor the supreme taste.
> One should experience the sensation of touch,
> Pursuing the five types of sense-objects.
>
> One will quickly become awakened ....[10]

East Asian Buddhist literature, drawing from the broader strains of the Daoist reverence of mountains, rivers, and trees, expresses a similar admiration of the physical and natural world, some seeing even rocks and grasses as infused with buddha-nature (LaFleur 1998).

The ethic of appreciation that has more recently become intertwined with Buddhist and Buddhist-derived meditative practices is, however, something new. It is part of the modern valorization of worldly life, what Charles Taylor calls the "affirmation of ordinary life." The idea is that the value and dignity of human life does not reside outside it but in the manner of living it. This includes things that would have been considered too mundane to be worthy of notice in earlier periods like labor, child-rearing, and production. The ordinary person, rather than the noble warrior or king, becomes the center of artistic attention in modern art and literature, where ordinary experience is valorized and, in some cases, even sacralized. Much of the multifaceted world of global, cosmopolitan late-modernity flows from the European Enlightenment, and one of its distinctive characteristics was a broad sense of world-affirmation. Most inheritors of this tradition have as part of their social imaginary a general sense that the world and worldly activity are goods in and of themselves. Marriage, reproduction, and work attain an esteem absent in medieval times, when the world was often considered a place of brief, temporary residence prior to occupying one's true home in the afterlife. The United States in particular has been the seat of a kind of world-affirming optimism, taking hold in the nineteenth century and characterized by a sense of progress, lack of limitation, the possibility of ever-increasing improvement of one's lot, and the unlimited improvability of society. Pleasure was positively reevaluated, as was material well-being. A positive view of the prospects of worldly satisfaction is, of course, by no means exclusive to the modern West, nor was it untempered by the unique horrors of the twentieth century, but it has been a prominent and enduring feature of the modern and late-modern eras (Taylor 1989, 211–304; also, in relation to modern Buddhism, see McMahan 2008, ch. 8).

Contemporary mindfulness practices have embedded themselves in this world-affirming ethos, absorbing it so thoroughly as to transform the significance of the practice itself. Consider a standard exercise in MBSR courses. One of the first things students do is eat a raisin. They first look at the raisin, notice its folds and contours, then eat it excruciatingly slowly, with complete focus on the flavors, sensations, textures—all the nuances of the experience of this simple, everyday activity. The exercise is designed to bring increased attention to something very familiar in order to uncover hidden dimensions of ordinary experience. The clear implication is that all experiences are like this. They all contain hidden aspects, secret delights, normally occluded subtleties to which we, in our mindless routines, have become blind. To increase attention to the fine-grained qualities of our ordinary experiences is to truly live our life rather than miss it in a haze of daydreams, distractions, and mental chatter. The underlying message is: the raisin is *good*; your sense-experience is *good*; your life as an embodied being who eats and digests and has sex and enjoys the sights, sounds, tastes, sensations, and smells of the natural world is *good*.

The purpose of close attention to the ordinary phenomena of embodied experience in the early Buddhist meditation texts is quite different. These practices are designed to bring about disenchantment (*nibbida*—sometimes translated "revulsion") with all phenomena and to develop dispassion (*viraga*) and detachment from them. There is still an element of detachment in the MBSR version: one detaches from one's ordinary habitual attitudes and mindless sleepwalking through life in order to discover the hidden treasures just below the surface. And it is not just treasures: sometimes one finds ugly emotions, hidden internal conflicts, repressed desires. But underlying it all is the idea that in order to deal with such difficulties, as well as appreciate the wonders of life, one must be mindful and increase one's scope of awareness—and that, ultimately, even in the face of old age, sickness, and death, embodied human life is good in and of itself, whether or not there is an afterlife or nirvana. The very fact that it is fleeting means one should cultivate *appreciation* for it.

Preparing the Way: Transcendentalism and Attentive Appreciation

The fabric of this reorientation of the contemplative attitude toward embodied experience and the material world was woven by a combination of threads from several Asian and European-American traditions. In addition to the affirmation of ordinary life and the shift toward world-affirmation, nineteenth-century Americans and Europeans began to cultivate the idea that focused and detailed attention to various facets of the world was spiritually nurturing. Attention to natural phenomena, for some, involved not just the objectifying analytical gaze of the sciences but also contemplation of the interface between the mind and the natural world, to the movements of the soul prompted by trees, animals, rivers, and mountains.

The Transcendentalists, along with other nineteenth-century thinkers, deserve special mention as preparers of a space for Buddhist and Hindu meditative practices in the West, as well as the transformation of these practices into exercises in this-worldly appreciation. This involved not only their intimate contemplations of the natural world but also their prescient scrutiny of attention itself. Even a century before Buddhist meditative practices took hold in North America, education reformers in New England began to create practices of cultivating attention in their students in response to new historical conditions that they believed harmed young minds. Urbanization, mass media, and the monotony of factory work, they contended, all created damage to the psyche that could be healed through harnessing the redemptive powers of attentiveness. According to Caleb Smith, this was a therapeutic project as well as an ethical one geared toward restoring agency and virtue that was being undermined by emerging industrialism. Such disciplines promised to "reshape character by establishing habits of watchfulness over the self" and "relieve the teacher of the work of surveillance" by "plac[ing] a mechanism of self-regulation inside students' minds," which one reformer called "*conscience or the inward voice*" (Smith 2019, 893. Italics original). Such disciplines were thought to be increasingly necessary for self-control and development of character in the modern, secularizing age.

Henry David Thoreau combined a new reverence for the natural world with an emphasis on cultivating heightened attentiveness in order to fully appreciate its salutary effects on the soul. Unlike the education reformers, however, who advocated cultivating attention in young minds for the sake of moral self-monitoring and conformity to social standards, Thoreau's arts of attentiveness were inseparable from his critique of the dominant emerging social forces of accelerating modernity, industrialism, and the increasing bureaucratization of ordinary life. For him, training attention in the observation of natural phenomena and the workings of the mind itself could potentially break the power of those dehumanizing forces. The education reformers sought to cultivate attention in the interest of training their students to discipline themselves and thereby become responsible citizens who could monitor themselves and conform to the dictates of the social order. Thoreau, in contrast, sought to harness attention as a way of breaking the grip of social control, power, and established authority, redeeming the human from what he saw as an increasingly mechanized society and its suppression of creative thought and inquiry. In Smith's analysis:

> The reformers want to cultivate submission, and Thoreau prefers to stir up disobedience, but they pursue these different projects by way of the same operation: isolating the self, extracting it from its entanglements in the social and material world, so that they can analyze, with an eye toward repairing, its relation to others and objects that now seem alien to it. Attention takes this new shape within secular history—as the dream of its transcendence. (Smith 2019, 903)

Disciplining the attention, "living deliberately," slowing down the pace of life to a crawl, allowing the minutiae of the world to enter the open gates of the senses was, for Thoreau, the antidote to an increasingly sick civilization.

Thoreau and his fellow Transcendentalists (as well as their intellectual cousins, the European Romantics) laid the foundations on which the Beat writers and the antiauthoritarian, countercultural figures would build when they inaugurated the widespread use of Buddhist meditation in America in the mid-to-late twentieth century. Their combination of disciplines of heightened attentiveness, valorization of nature, suspicion of social conformity, and resistance to authority provided much of the language into which Buddhist meditative practices would be translated. In many American and European articulations of these practices, the traditional Buddhist suspicion of the phenomenal world is displaced onto social institutions and authority. The ethic of appreciation turns the early Buddhist orientation toward the material world and the body on its head. That approach scrutinized and analyzed the processes of embodied experience in order to bring about disenchantment with them and to cultivate the conviction that these processes were inevitably tied to suffering and transience and, therefore, must be transcended. Modern meditation brings with it an ethic of appreciation that combines East Asian esteem of the natural world with the Romantic and Transcendentalist idea that close attention to nature, as well as the movements of the mind and heart, uncover hidden interior depths, truths, and delights. What is to be eschewed, on this model, are the social structures and external authority that would impose pregiven conceptions and values on this more raw, intimate experience.

The other dichotomy that gets turned on its head in the ethic of appreciation as applied to meditation is the Orientalist bifurcation of "East" and "West." The pervasive image of Asian cultures during the period of settler colonialism was, again, that the West was rational, technological, active, and masculine while the East was irrational, intuitive, passive, and feminine. The Transcendentalists were among the first Americans to begin to give a positive valuation to the latter set of characteristics and to imagine that Asian traditions may offer a reclamation of something that was being lost in the relentless drive toward technological progress and industrial production. This re-evaluation did not, of course, reach beyond these truncated and stereotyped images of East and West, and it opened the floodgates of the exotification and mystification of Asian culture that still persists today (Iwamura 2011). But it was historically important in that it prepared the way for an openness to Buddhist technologies of self that promised to plunge awareness beyond the confines of instrumental rationality and institutionally conditioned thinking to the interior depths that were a new fascination among Romantics and Transcendentalists, as well as their twentieth-century countercultural descendants.

Meditation in the Immanent Frame

Beyond just laying the foundations of incorporating the ethic of appreciation—of nature, of the body, of the senses, and of the intricate nuances of human experience—into Buddhist meditative practices, Thoreau and his fellow cultivators of attention left a more complex legacy. The tension between Thoreau's tying the arts of attention to an antiauthoritarian project and the education reformers' harnessing them to social conformity and cohesion presages debates about the uses of mindfulness today. Is mindfulness a felicitous tool for creating more productive workers to feed the system of global capital? Is it a way of keeping overworked employees slightly less anxious and more compliant during their 24/7 work weeks? Or does it focus the critical faculties of the mind for resistance against systems of routinization, commodification, and oppression? For critical inquiry into the social hierarchies and oppressive structures? Or for a day of immersion in the natural world away from the dehumanizing strain of the office? Or a relaxing destress after a hard day of protesting against such dehumanization? The early debates over the uses to which heightened attentiveness should be put laid down some of the parameters within which mindfulness continues to be understood today. The tension between meditation as an aid to conforming to social, professional, and cultural norms, on the one hand, and as an aid to questioning those norms, on the other, is baked into the fabric of secular adaptations of Buddhist meditation and is refracted across several ways of conceiving of what kind of ethical subject meditation helps to create.

No matter what uses mindfulness is put to today, they are most often this-worldly or aim at a kind of transcendence within immanence. Meditation teachers seldom encourage the cultivation of the desire to escape the world. Indeed, such a sentiment today carries a whiff of irresponsibility at a time of multiple social, political, and planetary crises. Instead, they might encourage acceptance of the aspects of the world that cannot be changed, aspiration to help the world and its living beings, and always—*appreciation* of the world and one's embodied life. The mindful savoring of food, the affirmation of the value of the body, the de facto assumption that immersion in nature not only removes distractions but also is healing and nurturing—all of these staples of modern meditation are not wholly unprecedented. They have antecedents in Tantra and East Asian Buddhisms. Nevertheless, the particular character they have acquired today represents something new—meditation as part of an ethic of appreciation within the broader social imaginary of modern secularism.

9
Meditation and the Ethic of Authenticity

> **Dispatches from the Worlds of Meditation: 9**
> The drive for authenticity is intrinsic to human nature. Meditation can help us recognize our unique place in the world by focusing our attention inwards without the distraction of thoughts or impulses. It can help us connect with our true, authentic self and act from a place of integrity.
> —From *Insight Timer*, "the #1 app for sleep, anxiety, and stress"[1]

Authenticity in Modern Western Thought

I sometimes ask my students if they have seen the movie in which two people from very different backgrounds—class, race, nationality, etc.—fall in love. The couple struggles through various obstacles conspiring to keep them apart, like the opposition of their families and friends and the norms of their society. After these external forces nearly tear them asunder, they follow their hearts and find a way to stay together, living happily ever after. What was the name of that movie? They laugh, realizing that they've seen many movies with that general plot. Then I ask if they've seen the one with a similar setup—different backgrounds, social obstacles, etc.—and in the end the two realize their folly and, for the sake of grandma, the boss, the village, the extended family, or the nation, they break up with their true love and go with the boring but more suitable mate. This film probably exists—maybe it's an arthouse dig at romantic comedies—but no one in the class has seen it.

The point is not about the relatively recent invention of romantic love but about the more general orientation of which it is a part. Countless cultural products affirm an understanding of authenticity that is generally seen, as the dispatch above affirms, as "intrinsic to human nature," but is actually historically and culturally particular. Books, movies, songs, and catchy phrases invite

Rethinking Meditation. David L. McMahan, Oxford University Press. © Oxford University Press 2023.
DOI: 10.1093/oso/9780197661741.003.0009

you to "be yourself," "find yourself," "actualize yourself." "You do you!" In the broadest sense, this orientation envisions individuals in their uniqueness in an antagonistic relationship to the surrounding cultural norms. Individuals are conceived as independent entities and society as a collection of the many unique individuals. One is not first a son or daughter, a member of a family, clan, or nation, but an individual with distinctive characteristics that demand recognition. In some accounts, this uniqueness is self-determined to some extent; in others, it is discovered within, after which it becomes a moral imperative to be true to oneself, that is, to be *authentic*. Although this orientation comes to us from a lineage of philosophers and literary figures, popular versions have become pervasive enough in the United States that they can be condensed in an "inspirational quote card." And they have. One by Emily McDowell that has gone viral includes this:

> Your true self is right there, buried under cultural conditioning, other people's opinions, and inaccurate conclusions you drew as a kid that became your beliefs about who you are. "Finding yourself" is actually returning to yourself. An unlearning, an excavation, a remembering who you were before the world got its hands on you.

Meditation comes into the picture as a way of either discovering or creating this authentic identity. In order to be authentic, according to professor of social work and best-selling motivational author, Brené Brown, we must, with the help of mindfulness, "let go of who we think we're supposed to be and embrace who we really are."[2] Authenticity, as this language suggests, implicitly pits the individual against external forces of tradition, social norms, and expectations and affirms the need to assert one's unique individual desires, values, and sense of self. Authenticity becomes an *ethic* in the sense that the demand to be true to oneself, even in the face of external pressures to the contrary, becomes an implicit moral imperative.

Sentiments like these are so pervasive today that they are taken as universal wisdom, and there is something that virtually all readers of this book likely embrace about them. But they would be quite out of place in many times and places. In a culture in which an *ethic of honor* based on birth predominates, for example, one might distinguish oneself by heroically upholding the values of one's proper station in life—the aristocracy or the knighthood. In Confucian-influenced societies the emphasis on shame, close family bonds, self-sacrifice for the collective good, and harmony between individuals and society has tempered the kind of individual-versus-society ethos that marks the ethic of authenticity in the West. In a casual sense, one might use the term "authentic" to indicate not being duplicitous—not deceiving others or, indeed, oneself. Or it might indicate something about culture: I might feel "inauthentic" doing the rituals of another culture because I cannot feel at home in them and perform them whole-heartedly. In a Buddhist context, for example, many westerners feel this way about chanting or doing full-body prostrations before a buddha-image or a teacher. Even these casual uses of the term arguably ride on the back of the more specific ethic of authenticity I am discussing here. And this ethic has a particular history. We need recount only a few highlights to understand the general trajectory and relevance to our subject of meditation and its relation to culture and society.

The European ideal of authenticity emerged in the seventeenth and eighteenth centuries as part of an increasing awareness of interiority, a sense of the unique inwardness of each individual, along with the political ideal of individual rights, that has marked the modern period. The source of morality, promotors of this ideal contended, is understood to reside in the interior of the individual person, in contrast to social norms and external authority. True morality—in contrast to mere calculation of advantage, conformity to exterior demands, or hope of divine reward and fear of punishment—comes from the independent voice within. Jean Jacques Rousseau, one of the ideal's early and most prominent advocates, insisted that morality consists in finding one's true, authentic voice within, which is too frequently obscured by the "passions" and by our dependence on others for guidance. The emergence of authenticity as an ethic also entailed a shift away from an ethic dominated by honor and sincerity. Hegel, for example, critiqued the ideal of the "sincere" person who, in his rendering, strives uncritically to embody the norms of his society. He saw such striving as preventing the emergence of individual consciousness and impeding the development of "spirit," which, in turn, entailed the maturing of autonomy strong enough to withstand external social norms (Golomb 1995).

While the ethic of authenticity originates within Christianity, its nonreligious espousers were quite influential in the twentieth century. Jean-Paul Sartre, for example, rejected any notion of a pregiven meaning to human life, which means that we are completely free to determine our interpretation of things, what significance events have, and what matters to us. Through these choices, moreover, we constitute ourselves. Authenticity in this sense means avoiding, as much as possible, "bad faith," deceiving ourselves by denying our freedom and the responsibility it entails, just going along with circumstances as if we had no choice (Sartre 1992 [1943], 710 ff.). Much of the discourse on authenticity emerges in reaction to the perceived "massification" (in

Kierkegaard's words) of society, the sense, in the industrial revolution and then in postindustrial societies, that human beings were becoming mere objects, cogs in a machine, and must assert a sense of agency and individuality in the face of the faceless and dehumanizing features of the modern world. In most historical contexts, "who am I?" and "what should I do?" have been questions mostly settled from birth. Within democratic contexts, settling these matters for oneself has emerged as a prominent ideal (one that, needless to say, still faces variable constraints based on class, race, gender, and socio-political circumstances). Charles Taylor calls the ideal of authenticity one of "self-determining freedom": "It is the idea that I am free when I decide for myself what concerns me, rather than being shaped by external influences. . . . Self-determining freedom demands that I break the hold of all such external impositions, and decide for myself alone" (1991: 27).

Edward Shils captures the flavor of the ideal and its implicit valorization of the individual over the collective (along with a bit of derision hinting at a common critique, which we will address later) from the perspective of a sociologist writing in the 1980s and characterizing a "deeper movement of mind in the past century":

> This is a metaphysical dread of being encumbered by something alien to oneself. There is a belief, corresponding to a feeling within each human being that there is an individuality lying in potentiality, which seeks an occasion for realization but is held in the toils of the rules, beliefs, and roles which society imposes. In a more popular, or vulgar, recent form, the concern "to establish one's identity," "to discover oneself," or "to find out who one really is," has come to be regarded as a first obligation of the individual. . . . They suggest that the real state of the self is very different from the acquired baggage which institutions like families, schools, and universities impose. To be "true to oneself" means . . . discovering what is contained in the uncontaminated self, the self which has been freed from the encumbrance of accumulated knowledge, norms, and ideals handed down by previous generations. (Shils 1981: 10–11)

The seeds of this ideal of authenticity were planted in the Enlightenment and Romanticism, and in the twentieth century developed further in Existentialism, humanistic psychology, and the Human Potential movement. And although these movements have faded, many of their ideals have embedded themselves in late-modern cultures, not just in Europe and North America, but now across the globe. It was inevitable that when Buddhist meditation began to appear in Europe and North America, it would be reinterpreted in the idiom of this ideal.[3]

Meditation and the Ethic of Authenticity

When Buddhist meditation began to enter the orbit of western thought, it was often interpreted as a way of penetrating the concealed, interior depths of the individual self, a way to get past the clamor of the crowd, the invasive voices of "society" to something more authentic—even pristine—within. As we've seen, some forms of Buddhism are in no way inimical to the idea of an interior, a priori perfection, even a "true self," within. The Mahāyāna idea of buddha-nature is an indispensable component of Chan/Zen traditions, for example. As we discussed in chapter 7, the strong form of the doctrine suggests not just the potential of all beings to become buddhas; it asserts that all beings are already fully awakened buddhas but don't realize their innate perfection because it is covered up by adventitious cognitive distortions and affective impurities. In Zen and other traditions affirming this ideal, meditation is not a matter of cultivating the character so much as discovering this hidden perfect buddha within. The European and American ethic of authenticity was a magnet that drew this idea and its associated practices into the sphere of western secular sensibilities. Although the conception of buddha-nature was different from the Romantic understanding of the authentic self—for one thing, buddha-nature is identical in everyone, not one's own unique individual essence—the ideas resonated enough so that Zen could be entwined with the modern quest for authenticity. It also accorded with the strains of European and American thought that affirmed the basic goodness of human nature. Rousseau's contention that human beings are naturally good but were inevitably corrupted by society worked its way through the Romantics and Transcendentalists and into humanistic psychology and the mid-to-late twentieth-century countercultural spiritual exploration that would help create a space for Asian meditative traditions in the West.

A few examples will suffice to show how meditation, particular Zen meditation, was interpreted along these lines. D. T. Suzuki, the most influential twentieth-century shaper of western perceptions of Zen, uses the language of the "unconscious" to describe this deep interior essence, the realization of which resolves all tension and anxiety: "Our limited consciousness, inasmuch as we know its limitation, leads us to all sort of worry, fear, unsteadiness. But as soon as it is realized that our consciousness comes out of something which, though not known in the way relative things are known, is intimately related to us, we are relieved of every form of tension and are thoroughly at rest and at peace with ourselves and with the world generally" (Suzuki 1960, 16–17). This unconscious deep within, according to Suzuki, is the source of all true creativity and is one's fundamental identity, but one requires special training to come into direct contact with it. For popularizers of Zen like Alan Watts, this deeper sense of self is more explicitly set up against the "social self." Watts portrays the process of awakening by the Zen meditator as one of getting beyond the "acquired self" or "ego," which is "that self he has believed himself to be [but which is] nothing but a pattern of habits or artificial reactions." One who is identified with this ego acts according to "socially conditioned habit . . . unconsciously acting his role, and not showing his original face." Only by overcoming this socially derived self can he come to the "original face" of the famous *kōan*, his true interior nature (which is, in turn, one with the nature of everything) (1973 [1958], 69–70). Picking up on the suspicion of institutions inherent in the ethic of authenticity, Watts suggests that Zen is capable of "overcoming cultural conditioning," because it (Zen) is not "institutionalized" and its "ancient exponents were 'universal individualists' " who did not rely on formal authority or organizations (a rather dubious assertion, by the way). Zen, according to William Barrett in an introduction to a collection D. T. Suzuki's of essays, "is individualistic, and so iconoclastic and antinomian in its individualism that it will seem irreverent to many Westerners; but this is only because Zen wishes to strip the individual naked in order to return him to himself" (1961, xviii–xix). Sheldon Kopp, in his popular 1972 book *If You Meet the Buddha on the Road, Kill Him!*, condenses the issue succinctly in his interpretation of the Chinese Chan master Linji's famous admonition:

> The Zen Master warns: "If you meet the Buddha on the road, kill him!"
> This admonition points up that no meaning that comes from outside of ourselves is real. The Buddhahood of each of us has already been obtained. We need only recognize it. Philosophy, religion, patriotism, all are empty idols. The only meaning in our lives is what we each bring to them. Killing the Buddha on the road means destroying the hope that anything outside of ourselves can be our master. (1972: 140)

These and other thinkers adapted Zen and other Buddhisms piecemeal into the vision of essentially good human beings alienated from their true, authentic nature by restrictive societal expectations and institutions. Meditation became a way of coming to a self-transparent, self-authorized truth within. The introjection into standardized models of mindfulness of the injunction to observe the mind *nonjudgmentally* (something, as we've seen, that is absent in many classical Buddhist accounts) likely is part and parcel of this adaptation to the ideal of authenticity. Judgement implies the internalized imposition of external, societal (and perhaps, more specifically, Christian and Jewish) evaluations on one's raw, authentic experience.

It was, in part, the magnetic pull of the ideal of authenticity that attracted selected anecdotes from Zen literature depicting the madcap antics of iconoclastic Zen masters befuddling their students with their unpredictable utterances and actions. And the authenticity magnet left behind much that did not fit into this ethic—the insistence on the authority of lineage, the militaristic discipline of the Zen monastery and its ubiquitous rituals. These anecdotes portray Zen masters as acting from an inscrutable certainty beyond social convention, impervious to doubt, hesitation, and anxiety. They spontaneously break the rules, even Buddhist ones (burning a buddha statue for warmth, "killing" buddhas, smacking their students, killing a cat, carrying a woman across a river despite vows not to touch women), in order to demonstrate their understanding. Seen through the lens of the ethic of authenticity, the Zen master did not act out of fidelity to an institution or doctrine but from an unshakable understanding of reality itself, discerned intuitively within the deep recesses of the individual mind and discovered through *zazen*. He was beyond rational calculation of advantage and disadvantage and acted spontaneously out of an intuitive reservoir of wisdom discovered deep within. He was, in other words, authentic.

Alienation and the Modern Meditator

The comingling of selected elements of Zen literature and the ethic of authenticity emerged in the context of the pervasive postwar sense of alienation. For many intellectuals of the time, alienation was the primary affliction of modern life, and it covered a variety of malaises. Marx's idea of the alienation of workers from their labor with the emergence of the dehumanizing and repetitive work of mass production in factories was a part of the story. But it took on more expansive connotations in the twentieth century. Martin Jay summarizes various accounts of alienation in this period this way:

> The prevailing assumption behind all of these accounts was that feeling estranged—whether from one's personal or communal identity, one's creations, or the human species as a whole—was a reason for profound dismay. Alienation could suggest, among other things, the domination of the subject by the object, the self by the other, the organic by the mechanical, and the living by the dead. Understood psychologically, socially, religiously or philosophically, it was a painful obstacle to feeling whole or at one with the world. Being settled in an identity and comfortable in one's skin were taken as preferable to being rootless, dispossessed or self-fractured. For the lucky few cosmopolitans, rootlessness might have meant being

at home everywhere—but for those who felt like permanent exiles, it meant being at home nowhere. (Jay 2018)

Is it a coincidence that Zen, which gained traction in the West during the age of alienation, promised to guide practitioners to their "true home"? Mid-twentieth-century western authors frequently held out the hope that Zen was a way toward recovering a lost wholeness and overcoming the sense of disenchantment, fragmentation, nihilism, anxiety, and alienation keenly felt in intellectual and artistic circles at the time. For Watts, Zen provided a "way of recognizing and dissolving the conflict or contradiction of self-consciousness" (1973 [1958], 67). The awakened Zen master is a "completely natural man" who has a "complete absence of inner conflict" and is "never caught in the vicious cycles of anxiety or indecisive doubt," and is "possessed of complete inner freedom" (67–8). In the face of pervasive alienation, uncertainty, and doubt, as well as loss of confidence in social institutions, meditation promised a way to a kind of self-authenticating certainty within.

It is worth pointing out what is specific about the ethic of authenticity and what is unique about its modern articulation: it sets up a duality between a person's social masks and something more authentic to be discovered within. Granted, this may resemble features of premodern interpretations of the dynamics of meditation. Advaita Vedānta philosophers insist on an ultimately real self (*ātman*), the "inner controller" (*antaryamin*), in comparison to which all other attributions of selfhood, including caste, lineage, body, and one's ordinary sense of "I," are illusory. In Tathāgatha-garbha thought, buddha-nature, again, is often described as a "buddha within," a pre-existent awakened nature that is obscured by the impurities of distorting concepts and misguided emotions. Nevertheless, these traditions do not present the sacred interior in direct contrast to one's alienated social roles, the way modern accounts do. True, the Buddha is represented as someone who left his inherited social role to find a profound truth within; however, Buddhist doctrine does not suggest that what is ultimately to be overcome to reach awakening is primarily external, societal influence but rather past karmic predispositions and adventitious mental impurities. The idea, moreover, of awakening as a purely personal affair has some resonance with Buddhist ideas. No doubt, meditation literature tends to venerate the lone ascetic; nevertheless, the role of the teacher and community has always been considered essential. For all of the iconoclastic rhetoric of Zen literature, in practice, even the most profound meditative experiences are authenticated by the Zen master. The incorporation of the Buddhist meditation and buddha-nature into the modern, more individualistic, ethic of authenticity, therefore, yields a novel configuration.

Evaluating the Ethic of Authenticity

To help clarify the stakes of the ethic of authenticity for Buddhist meditation, let's consider a few critiques of the ethic, which has come under scrutiny and criticism in recent decades. Meditative approaches that have become entwined with the modern project of authenticity are subject to these critiques as well. One critique takes us back to the point I've been arguing throughout the book: that meditation is more social and cultural than it is often represented, and that it is always embedded in a social and cultural context with a variety of ideals, concepts, and values that shape meditative experiences as well as the purposes to which meditative practices are put. That doesn't mean that through meditation one cannot break through to profound personal insights or have novel experiences that are not completely prefigured by one's cultural repertoires. It does mean, however, that a lot happens on the way that is deeply culturally conditioned, and even such breakthroughs are advancements beyond a particular, socially embedded conceptual-affective configurations to *other* such configurations—a point that I will develop further in the next two chapters. The contention that meditation is primarily about having purely private, sui generis mental experiences issuing from a realm untainted by the social and cultural is dubious.

This is essentially a philosophical point about how human beings are constituted, one that resonates with recent critiques of the idea of a pure, transparent interior self set over against external objects and social forces. Such critiques are widespread, from thinkers such as Theodor Adorno, Michel Foucault, and Richard Rorty, as well recent analyses of consciousness in cognitive science and embodied cognition. Authenticity, on these accounts, rests on the flawed idea of a singular self or stream of experience that can be thoroughly transparent to interior inspection. It neglects the degree to which "selves" are constituted by what is "not self," by imitation of others and embeddedness in social imaginaries. Indeed, the very idea of being true to oneself, paradoxically, is deeply cultural and historically constituted. Modern society demands that you flout social expectations, think for yourself, and be true to yourself—and there are many established cultural forms for doing so, from wearing goth clothing to becoming a "disruptor" in Silicon Valley.

The thrust of these ideas is that meaning is not created solely within in self-authenticating, private acts; it is a social process embedded in (though, again, not wholly determined by) culture and its repertoires of ideas, aesthetics, tastes, and habits of mind. Philosophers in recent decades have been suspicious of, in Martin Jay's words, the idea of "the universal, knowing human subject which sat at the heart of traditional humanism. Proponents doubted that we could grasp a 'reality' unfiltered by culture and language. And if there were no access to reality without the welter of linguistic ambiguities and differences, it must also be impossible to bridge the gap between consciousness and being, thought and its objects, humans and the world they had created" (Jay 2018). Cognitive science has also become quite skeptical of any model of the self as a pure, interior individual author of thought and action in favor of a modular model in which cognition and behavior are the products of a complex network of associated processes, many of which are unconscious. These critiques resonate in some respects with the Buddhist skepticism about a static, independent self, though Buddhism is certainly more optimistic about the possibility of grasping "reality unfiltered by culture and language."

Another reservation about authenticity, and by association meditative practices interpreted through its lens, is what we might call a socioethical critique. The sociologist Christopher Lasch famously articulated this critique in his phrase "the culture of narcissism" (1991 [1979]). The worry is that, aside from whether it is *possible* to have the kind of self-transparency, certainty, and independent autonomy to which the ethic of authenticity aspires, the very aspiration is too self-centered and has deleterious effects on society. It is adjacent to a pervasive emphasis on self-fulfillment that implies, in his view, a degraded ability to recognize ethical demands external to efforts at one's own self-actualization. It might weaken social bonds and diminish empathy if it simply reduces the role of others to instrumental means to one's own self-fulfilling ends. This may contribute to disengagement with social and political realities and might even be deleterious to democracy itself, which presupposes citizen engagement. It also may lead to a kind of atomism and social isolation that sociologists argue are increasing in postindustrial societies (Putnam 2000). Finally, it rests on what Robert Bellah has called "ontological individualism," the conviction that human beings are fundamentally independent and separate beings to whom sociality is essentially compromising, unnatural, and alienating from one's true nature (Bellah et al. 1985, Trilling 1972, Guignon 2004).

Meditative practices entwined with modern spiritualities emphasizing self-fulfillment and personal growth exclusive to broader social concerns have come under similar critical scrutiny. An understanding of meditation as aiming primarily at individual authenticity suggests that mindfulness is a tool for attaining whatever personal goals one happens to have. Anything that challenges one's personal vision may be discarded. Excised from the comprehensive ethical and philosophical worldview of Buddhism, it might foster a kind of liberalism of neutrality that carries no particular values except what is decided by individual practitioners in the fulfillment of their goals. At its most banal, mindfulness might become simply another instrument of narcissism, an accoutrement of developing a superficial, atomistic identity, an aid to "lifestyle enhancement" rather than a practice of deep critical self-inquiry. Moreover, discovering oneself in the age of social media is almost inevitably mediated through commercial interests that monetize and commodify countless tools for constructing identity, from clothes to gadgets to, indeed, mindfulness itself. Or, a parallel concern, mindfulness may create a passive, spectatorial mode of disengagement with broader social and political realities beyond the self.[4]

There is another side to this issue, however. Some thinkers argue that the versions of authenticity subject to some of these critiques may be something of a caricature of the earlier impetus of the ethic of authenticity. Indeed, several have attempted to rehabilitate the ethic, and this discussion also tracks with more recent trends in the understanding of meditation as socially relevant. Charles Taylor has argued that the narcissistic versions of authenticity are actually distortions of the ideal, and the idea that "one must break free of all such external impositions and decide for oneself alone" is not a necessary part of authenticity (1991, 27). What is important for anyone, he contends, is necessarily based on a collectively constituted notion of the good that requires negotiation and maintenance in collaboration with others. In democratic societies in which one's identity is not wholly fixed, as it would be in, say, a feudalistic one, one's own authenticity and identity, in fact, requires the recognition of others in order to be meaningful. A more viable ideal of authenticity, then, involves committing to a notion of the good that is not simply one's own self-discovered possession but a matter of collective questioning and democratic negotiation. In a similar vein, Charles Guignon suggests that authenticity need not be synonymous with self-absorption but is, to the contrary, only possible in a "free society," and thus it carries with it obligations to sustain and nurture that society's well-being. This can only happen through being clear and committed to one's desires and convictions in the democratic arena (Guignon 2004). In a similar vein, recent expositors of meditation have insisted that it is not just a means for private self-fulfillment and enrichment but can be an aid to thinking deeply, clarifying one's commitments, and mobilizing these commitments not only in the personal but also in the social and political arena.

We have been focusing on how Buddhist and Buddhist-derived meditation practices have become entwined with the modern, western discourse of authenticity, and the idea that meditation might get the practitioner to her own authentic insights and foster self-determining action in the world. This is a largely secular interpretation of the purpose of meditation, one that takes for granted liberal ideas of the self-determination, self-discovery, and self-actualization of individuals combined with the aspiration to freedom from external constraints. Such ideals are nearly inescapable in the contemporary world, and they cannot simply be written off. After all, without such ideals, it would be hard to argue for the self-determination of women, minorities, and LGBTQ people. But such freedoms, many theorists argue, cannot be understood in an abstract or absolute sense but must address the particularities of different societies and cultural contexts. A coherent account of meditation can, likewise, offer the promise of reflexive inquiry, self-discovery, and self-creation within the constraints and configurations of particular cultural contexts—even while proffering the prospect of expanding beyond their limitations. In the next two chapters, we will develop some of these possibilities.

The Real Thing

A final note on authenticity: as Buddhist traditions become more fully understood in the West, some practitioners become more concerned with authenticity in an altogether different sense than that of the ethic we've been discussing. They are concerned with practicing the *authentic* Dharma, with its promise of genuine awakening as understood by Buddhist traditions and handed down generation to generation. It is becoming more widely understood in Buddhist circles in the West that the meditative traditions they have learned have been tailored to modern western ideas and predilections. For some, this understanding fosters a desire to get back to a more "authentic" Buddhism and shed the innovations that have accrued in recent decades. "*It's bullshit!*" declares an American Zen monk, Jiryu Mark Rutschman-Byler, to his California teacher in his book, *Two Shores of Zen*:

> I'm not just complaining. He needs to meet me, to understand that I'm tired of this American Buddhist "Upper Middle Way." I'm tired of the sexual dramas, the talk of "income streams" and "personnel costs." I don't want any more of the peanut butter that's refilled in the snack area as quickly as it's used. I don't want a snack area, period. The great monks of old didn't have a "snack area," much less one stocked with blueberry-tofu-cashew smoothies and leftover chocolate cake.... But I'm frustrated, and I'm tired, and it's dawning on me, like a slow, unstoppable train, that if I'm really serious about this Buddhism thing, I may well need to abandon this California imitation of it. I don't mean to disparage the Sangha, my peers and my teachers, but I have vowed to end all suffering, my own and others'. And I've glimpsed the possibility of that kind of salvation, but the lifestyle here is not

pushing me to take the plunge, to realize the one final truth that will shatter all delusions and liberate all beings. (2009, 18–19, italics original)

After this conversation, Rutschman-Byler indeed takes the plunge and takes his quest for authentic Zen to Japan, where he practices in Japanese monasteries for two years.

Such aspirations to "traditional authenticity," however, produce their own paradoxes, as he finds out. The "authentic" Zen of Japan was adapted from China and has gone through dramatic transformations over many centuries. Vipassanā meditation, notwithstanding claims that it goes directly back to the Buddha, is a recent movement, born of colonial resistance and reconfigured to modern lay life (Braun 2013). Even the earliest Buddhist texts were compiled centuries after the life of Siddhārtha Gautama and bear clear traces of interpolation and adaptation to later circumstances. Scholars don't agree even about the Buddha's historical existence, let alone which ideas and utterances in the Pali suttas likely originated with him. Every teacher today insisting that their Buddhism or their meditative practices are "traditional" or "original" inevitably must reconstruct this "tradition" to some extent as a reaction to the "modern." There is no access to a primordially pure, original tradition, untainted by the interpretations of people situated in particular times and places. No resolution exists to this tension but a continuing, collective negotiation between the demands of fidelity to unique individual experience, emphasized in western articulations of the Dharma, and fidelity to more distinctively Buddhist training and conceptions of awakening found in classical accounts.

Contemporary seekers have produced a steady stream of books and articles about their attempts to shed westernized versions of Buddhism and inhabit the "authentic" Buddhism of Japan, Tibet, or Burma. Some, no doubt, have succeeded in some measure, but many accounts reveal just how deeply embedded practitioners are in their "home" cultural contexts, no matter how hard they try to slough them off. Indeed, it is common to hear or read that, ultimately, practitioners from California, London, or Sydney found that they could not "authentically" embody the traditions in their Asian contexts and were left to renegotiate a compromise. In Rutschman-Byler's case, he finds in Japan opportunities for deep, rigorous practice but also a Zen tradition in decline, with its own politics and limitations, itself influenced by western philosophy; one that fails, unsurprisingly, to live up to his idealistic hopes. He finally returns to his home sangha with only a slightly grudging acquiescence to his westernized Dharma.

Whichever path is better, or more traditional, or more conducive to real spiritual understanding and compassion, the basic fact that I'm left with is that simply I am a Western Buddhist, and that try as I might, my . . . Western Buddhist values underlie my practice. I have tried, and failed, to force myself to think that monastic practice is better than, or finally even necessary at all for meaningful, everyday worldly practice. Have I lost anything in that? Yes. Have I gained something?—indeed, my whole life, just as it is, reclaimed and renewed as precisely the territory of unsurpassed enlightenment. (182–3)

The demand for authenticity may be part of the inescapable fabric of modern social imaginaries. Whether in its hyperindividualized iterations, its more sociable versions, or its longing for ancient truths and lost ways of life, it speaks to the need for agency, self-determination, and self-responsibility that is a tacitly assumed good in contemporary life. Like the other tensions we have explored so far, the ones surrounding authenticity—between individual experience and authoritative tradition, between personal insight and collective wisdom—are not altogether alien to premodern iterations of Buddhism. And they cannot be considered separate from specific ideas of freedom, autonomy, and liberation, both in ancient Buddhist and modern secular meditative traditions. The next two chapters, therefore, consider these issues, both historically and philosophically.

10
Meditation and the Ethic of Autonomy

Dispatches from the Worlds of Meditation: 10
So freed! So thoroughly freed am I!—
from three crooked things set free:
from mortar, pestle,
& crooked old husband.
Having uprooted the craving
that leads to becoming,
I'm set free from aging & death.
                            —Muttā, in the *Therīgāthā*, verses of elder nuns, I.11.[1]

Introducing Autonomy

This poem, found in an early Indian collection of verse by Buddhist nuns, weaves together seamlessly and provocatively the two senses in which the Dharma has traditionally understood freedom. The last line celebrates the ultimate goal of the Buddhist path, liberation from rebirth in *saṃsāra*, the transcendence of time itself in the permanent bliss of nirvana. It celebrates the promise of freedom from all conditions of human embodiment. Yet Buddhist traditions have always been concerned with this-worldly well-being too, including at least some forms of freedom in a more mundane sense. In this case, the poem begins with a more immanent liberation attained upon joining the monastic sangha: freedom from the traditional domestic duties of a woman and from the nearly sacred role expected of a woman in ancient India, that of a devoted wife. It's hard to tell which freedom she's more excited about.

Buddhist and other Indian-originated meditative traditions have long been presented as practices of freedom and liberation. Perhaps it was inevitable that modern discourses of freedom, personal autonomy, and agency would be magnets for attracting them and that classical liberatory ideals would become intertwined with modern conceptions of personal and collective freedom. What we might call the *ethic of autonomy* is deeply embedded in modern societies, and its logic has governed how people think of themselves as individual

Rethinking Meditation. David L. McMahan, Oxford University Press. © Oxford University Press 2023.
DOI: 10.1093/oso/9780197661741.003.0010

and political actors. So in order to understand modern iterations of Buddhist meditation, we must examine how this ethic has drawn meditation into its orbit and shaped how people today think of meditative practices as conducive to freedom. This pervasive ethic, which overlaps in many ways with the ethic of authenticity, has played a powerful role in filtering, augmenting, and transforming the various meanings of meditation today, reimagining them in terms of modern, secular conceptions of freedom and the pervasive ideology of liberalism. Some versions of secular meditation interpret it in terms of classical liberal autonomy, which emphasizes the rational free choice of individuals. More recently, though, interpretations of meditation have arisen in conjunction with critiques of this conception. Each of these has a different understanding of the kind of autonomy meditation provides: the first, which I will call the Inner Citadel model, emphasizes developing a kind of invulnerable peace, certitude, and autonomy derived solely from within. The second, which I will call the Situated Autonomy model, stresses autonomy in particular contexts and emphasizes interdependence over individualism; it is also more open to social and political applications of meditation. In this chapter, I continue the philosophical-theoretical argument about the "work" that meditation does that I began in the first few chapters. Specifically, I will argue that the situated autonomy model makes more sense as a way to understand that work and the ways it might be conducive to an enhanced sense of agency. In the next chapter, I will continue this line of inquiry with a discussion of the concept of affordances and how it might be useful in developing a theoretical account of the role of meditation in enhancing situated autonomy. We begin, however, where we have already begun, expanding on Muttā's joyous exaltation of freedom, briefly sketching the sense of freedom, both this-worldly and otherworldly, suggested in the early Buddhist meditative literature.

Freedom in Classical Buddhism

In classical Buddhist literature, meditative practices were usually geared toward transcendent freedom, but, as we have discussed, they also served immanent purposes. The ultimate goal of *parinirvāṇa*—nirvana after death—entails freedom from rebirth, *saṃsāra*, and essentially all limitations whatsoever. It is said to be so utterly beyond worldly conditions that it is ultimately unthinkable from "this shore." But meditation has also been thought to grant a level of immanent freedom not available to the ordinary, worldly nonmeditator. Nirvana in this world is freedom from greed, hatred, and ignorance in one's everyday activities. It is said to grant freedom from bondage to destructive desires and emotional states. Meditative training will not free one from being shot by an arrow, but it can free one from inflicting yet a second "arrow" of "sorrow, grieving, and lamenting"—of compounding one's suffering by another layer of "mental" pain (*cetasikañca*) (SN 36.6). Precise awareness of the unfolding processes of the mind brings these processes to more explicit consciousness and reveals the ultimate illusoriness of the conceptual unities on which the destructive emotions are based. This allows for ethical freedom as conceived in Buddhist literature, i.e., the freedom born of meticulously observing the way thoughts, emotions, and impulses develop, and thus gaining more control over the process. The twentieth-century Burmese Vipassana teacher, Sayadaw U Pandita, encapsulates the classical understanding of the relationship between meditation and ethics:

> Moral restraint is not possible without the practice of *satipaṭṭhāna* [the establishment of mindfulness], as it is the power of observation that keeps the mind in control, to know what is suitable and what isn't; when knowledge develops, one makes the correct choices in life, knowing what is beneficial and what isn't. When the practice is undertaken meticulously together with ardent effort, one's mind can be purified, sheltered from hindrances and defilements. (U Pandita, 2016: 22)

Such precise observation also entails a kind of freedom born of knowledge that is said to dissolve the sense of oneself as a static, independent, and enduring entity, revealing instead the person as a complex of interdependent processes constituted by past actions (*karma*), as well as external factors. Becoming free from delusions of independent, static entities by "penetration" into their illusory nature, in turn, frees one to act in the world for the benefit of others and for one's own ultimate liberation. The monk who has mastered his meditation is autonomous in that he is said to be in complete control of his own mind.

> He thinks any thought he wants to think, and doesn't think any thought he doesn't want to think. He wills any resolve he wants to will, and doesn't will any resolve he doesn't want to will. He has attained mastery of the mind with regard to the pathways of thought.
>
> (AN 4.35)[2]

A great deal of classical Buddhist literature promises such internal freedom, both in the sense of being free *from* internal obstacles and causes of suffering and being free *to* think, act, and feel as one chooses. Such freedom is essential not only to achieving liberation but also to acting skillfully and ethically in the world.

Meditation and Modern Conceptions of Freedom

Several years ago, I interviewed some meditators in Sri Lanka and North America, asking, among other things, why they meditate and what they get out of the practice. One Sri Lankan forest monk—whose tiny hut I had to hike several miles into the forest outside of Kandy to find, but whom I originally found on Facebook—reiterated something very close to U Pandita's classical understanding of Buddhist meditation. It allowed one to observe one's mind, establish self-control, free oneself from destructive desires and emotions, and gradually purify the mind. The Americans were practitioners of Zen, Vipassana, or Tibetan traditions. Gary, a Zen practitioner of over twenty years, found relief from work and family stress and aspired to a state of "composure, tranquility, and resolve" that doesn't depend on "external circumstances." He was inspired by the famous story of the Zen master in feudal Japan who casually refuses to show deference to a military general who, offended and reaching for his sword, shouts: "Don't you realize you are standing before a man who could run you through without blinking an eye?" To which the master replies: "And do you realize that you are standing before a man who can be run through without blinking an eye?" Gary said that he strives to get beyond ambivalence, indecisiveness, and fear, to trust his instincts and to bring the unperturbed state of mind he sometimes feels during *zazen* to all situations. He insisted that meditation shows him that the only true source of happiness is within, and he therefore strives not to let his well-being depend on others or on contingent circumstances.

Shira, an experienced middle-aged Vipassana practitioner, said she meditates to calm down when her children are being difficult, to focus when she is scattered at work, to stop and tune in to what she referred to as "the big picture" in the midst of her hectic life. Even though meditation is a personal, inward experience, she insisted that it has brought her closer to her family and allowed her to be more engaged and focused in her work and more connected to the world around her. She feels that meditation has helped her to overcome psychological barriers to doing the things she really wants to do in her life. It has aided her in overcoming social anxiety and has been pivotal at times in clarifying her morals and goals. She is actively involved in a group that promotes legislation to fight climate change and says that her meditation is an essential element in her activism. It reminds her of the fragility and interconnectedness of all of life and of the immense suffering that climate change might produce for innumerable living beings.

The Americans—and even, to a lesser extent, the Sri Lankan monks I spoke with—brought to their practice underlying philosophical notions that entwine classical Buddhist ideas with modern, western conceptions of the individual, freedom, and autonomy. These orientations draw upon long-standing tensions in Buddhist traditions between striving for a private, imperturbable peace within and compassionate action in the world for the benefit of sentient beings—more broadly, between "other-worldly" and "this-worldly" aspirations. The axis of these two interpretations of meditation highlights some tensions in contemporary meditation as well: between individualized versions that emphasize internal peace of mind and psychological invulnerability to external events and influence, on the one hand, and those that emphasize interconnectedness, bringing the focus and clarity produced by meditation to particular this-worldly projects, including social and political freedom, on the other.

There is no one model today for conceiving of how meditation might be conducive to freedom and enhancement of human agency, but there are, I propose, these two broad countervailing tendencies. I treat these not necessarily as well-thought-out theoretical positions but, instead, general orientations on the ground that are worked out in individual meditation groups and essays in popular magazines more than in academic work.

The Inner Citadel Model

On this model meditative practices set up an interior space of invulnerability to external influence, thus allowing freedom to choose, decide, and act for oneself. The role of meditation in ethical agency on this model is that it is a means to actualize interior freedom—a freedom from social conditioning and identification with one's social roles—in order to choose the ethical path found within after deep investigation, analysis, and/or intuition. Moral imperatives are self-discovered, not derived from "society," dogma, institutions, or external sources.

The Situated Autonomy Model

This model offers a more contextual notion of freedom and ethical agency as embodied, embedded in social contexts, and systemically intertwined with other individuals, social institutions, and political structures. It sees social roles and identities as conditioned and limited, but recognizes that they still inform life in the world and must be addressed. The role of meditation in ethical agency on this model is that it helps to clarify one's position within the multiple, nested social and political contexts in which everyone is inevitably embedded, and helps one act intentionally on one's commitments within these contexts.

These are in some measure exaggerated, idealized representations. It is likely that few practitioners of contemporary meditation adhere to one model exclusively; rather, in practice, they are combined in various ways. Neither is wholly exclusive of the other, and in any meditator's lived experience they may overlap. But this particular tension seems to underlie some fundamental tendencies, interpretations, and debates present in contemporary meditation. Perhaps they constitute a spectrum of possibilities that individuals and groups combine and configure in a variety of unique ways.

My argument here is both historical and theoretical, addressing Buddhist meditation as it migrated to the West. Regarding the historical part, the Inner Citadel model emerged first, in the mid-to-late twentieth century, and was an important part of the initial alloying of Buddhist meditative practices and secular forms of life in the West (and later, globally). Several "magnets" in modern western intellectual and cultural life have drawn Buddhist meditation into the secular conceptions of autonomy, including dominant understandings of personal autonomy, postwar concerns with conformity, and countercultural, libertine attitudes.

The Situated Autonomy model is more recent and emphasizes modern iterations of Buddhist concepts of interdependence. It has gradually taken shape as a counterresponse to the individualism inherent in the Inner Citadel model and as part of the penetration of meditative practices into diverse domains of life—family, work, art, activism. It has focused less on solely internal and individualistic freedom and more on interdependence and ethical responsibility in a tight-knit world. It is more inclined to acknowledge human frailty and complexity, less beholden to the quest for invulnerability and certainty, and more amenable to social and political engagement. Both of these models are this-worldly in the sense that they are concerned primarily with cultivating ways of life in this world rather than ultimate transcendence of the world.

Liberalism and the Autonomous Self

The magnetic forces drawing Buddhist meditation into the discourses of the vast and plural tradition of modern western liberalism were the Romantic and Transcendentalist notions of freedom and authenticity (addressed in the last chapter), Enlightenment-influenced conceptions of liberty and self-governance, and postwar renewal of efforts to combat conformity and blind obedience to authority. All of these involved variations on the theme that each person is an autonomous individual or should aspire to be one. The dominant conception of freedom in the modern West involves freedom from being controlled by others, but many liberal theorists also emphasized that to be truly free one must be master of oneself as well. One can only be free if one is self-directed, or autonomous. According to the influential theorist Thomas Hill Green (1836–1882), if one is dominated by one's own uncontrollable impulses, one is not truly free, but is "in the condition of a bondsman who is carrying out the will of another, not his own" (1986 [1895]: 228). One is free if one can determine the shape of one's life, refuses to mindlessly follow custom, and can reflect and act on what one truly wants. This ideal of "positive liberty" amounted to freedom as self-control; one not only must be free from mere impulses and appetites in order to do what one truly desires, one must also be free to choose or discover one's own moral imperatives. As Rousseau put it: "For the impulse of appetite alone is slavery, and obedience to the law one has prescribed for oneself is freedom" (Rousseau, 283).

The narrative of the modern self, the cornerstone of which was personal autonomy, began at least in the seventeenth century. Conceptions of personal autonomy that developed among the philosophers of the Enlightenment, Romanticism, and Utilitarianism have become part of the default intuitions of many in the contemporary world, not just in the West. Often this constellation of ideas is described as "liberalism," though the notion of liberal freedom in the West is plural and contested (Laidlaw 2014, 142 ff.). For our purposes it is only necessary to highlight a few salient features of these conceptions to suggest how they have influenced contemporary understandings of how meditation is conducive to freedom, autonomy, and heightened agency.

The dominant concepts of autonomy and ethics were formulated by various Enlightenment thinkers, but Immanuel Kant provides a paradigmatic example. Kant presents reason as the capacity that secures sound moral decisions, while emotions cloud judgment and obscure the truth. As with the ethic of authenticity, the ability to secure moral autonomy rests, in part, with being capable of transcending cultural norms in order to discover one's own moral imperatives. Autonomy rests on independence, reliance on one's own reasoning, and the ability to think for oneself and come to one's own conclusions unswayed by social forces and emotional bonds, which compromise objectivity and undermine commitment to moral duty. Rational analysis and free choice are what secure moral capacity to act against ingrained habits and socially derived dispositions. In developing the capacities of reason, one achieves freedom from the passions and emotions that distort objectivity. In less rationalistic versions of liberalism, such as that of the Transcendentalists, reason was dethroned but, famously, the emphasis on personal independence and self-reliance remained.

These general conceptions of autonomy provided the ground in which the seeds of Buddhist meditation would be planted in the West in the twentieth century, when a more specific and urgent version of the idea of the autonomous subject was emerging. Although a handful of people in Europe and North America practiced Buddhist meditation in the late nineteenth and early twentieth centuries, these practices did not enter the West in a serious way until the postwar period, a time in which a newly energized individualism and emphasis on self-responsibility was prominent among psychologists and social thinkers. Many such thinkers were stunned by catastrophic rise of fascism in Germany, the mystery of how such a thing could have happened in the center of European culture, and the acquiescence of so many ordinary Germans to the demands of the Third Reich. Theorists like Theodor Adorno, as well as psychologists such as Erich Fromm, made vigorous efforts to analyze and find antidotes to herd mentality and mindless conformity, scrutinizing the processes that could distinguish the self-responsible ethical conscience from the clamor of the crowd and the demands of authority. Experiments showing how easily people conformed to social pressure became *de rigueur* in psychology and sociology textbooks. Recall Solomon Asch's famous experiments in which subjects in a group were asked to identify which lines on an illustration were longer and which were shorter. A surprising number affirmed with the majority in the room—who, unbeknownst to them, were collaborators with the researchers—that shorter lines were longer and longer lines were shorter, even though it was obvious that they were otherwise. Other illustrative studies include the infamous Milgram experiments, which attempted to ascertain the willingness of subjects to obey an authority figure asking them to administer (unbeknownst to them, fake) electric shocks to people (also collaborators) to measure "negative reinforcement on learning a task." As is well known, a surprising number of subjects were willing to "shock" the "learners" even when they appeared to be in great pain and even mortal danger.

The underlying motivation for such efforts was the desire to understand how to educate self-responsible individuals unwilling to conform to society's demands and to resist authority when it demanded unethical behavior. This desire to establish the foundations of an autonomous moral human being no doubt influenced the way meditation was interpreted and refashioned beyond Asia in the postwar era as an interior arena of the cultivation of personal choice, freedom, and responsibility. Indeed, some thinkers involved in the project of fostering greater individual autonomy, like Erich Fromm, were instrumental in popularizing meditation, especially Zen, combining it with psychology and enlisting it in the quest for personal autonomy (Fromm 1960). Thus Buddhist meditative practices were beginning to be conceived as possible means to the kinds of freedom conceived in the modern West.

Enlightenment rationalism and the more recent postwar effort to secure moral autonomy are just two varieties of modern western conceptions of autonomy, but they should suffice for our purposes. We have already addressed in the last chapter conceptions of freedom and authenticity rooted in Romanticism. These tendencies were expanded in the mid-to-late twentieth-century counterculture, during which Buddhist meditation was often interpreted as a way of achieving a kind of transgressive freedom, untainted by a decadent, postwar consumerist, materialist, and increasingly artificial culture.

The Inner Citadel of the Mind

To some extent, the gravitational pull of these pervasive western views of personal autonomy on Buddhist meditation makes sense. Classical accounts of meditation, though they reject an atomistic self, often emphasize training for an unaffected, nonattached mode of being in the world, one that emphasizes independence from the pull of family relationships, emotional entanglements, and social and political engagement. And, although Buddhist accounts do not enthrone reason as the sine qua non of moral autonomy, many recommend detached, reflexive self-scrutiny that overlaps in some respects with Enlightenment models of rational self-examination and moral reflection. The liberal ideal of "positive liberty" also resonates with aspects of the Buddhist conceptions of freedom in that it requires freedom from cravings and compulsions in order to be capable of acting on one's moral principles. Perhaps one difference is that Buddhist treatments of freedom do not insist that these principles *themselves* should be self-determined—rather the principles are derived from the Dharma, the Buddha's teachings on how things are and how one should act.

As the various Buddhist and western conceptions of freedom have become interlaced, a certain notion of autonomy has emerged in standardized versions of mindfulness, one that combines elements of the Buddhist and modern liberal conceptions of freedom. According to this model, the flurry of thoughts, emotions, desires, and ruminations that constitute so much of our experience is essentially unreal or leads us to false conclusions about ourselves, other people in our lives, and the world. These fleeting thoughts and feelings crystalize into fixed ideas and ingrained emotional patterns. We act, or rather, react, mechanically to this flurry (and the reactions themselves constitute part of the flurry), and thus become trapped in net of binding mental patterns. Mindfulness allows one to step back from the flurry, calm it down, observe it in a detached manner, and recognize its essential illusoriness, thus freeing oneself from identifying with it and being determined by it. This freedom *from* interior bonds also entails freeing oneself *to* act deliberately and intentionally—or in some accounts, spontaneously—and to choose one's thoughts and emotions, that is, not so much choose which ones to experience (surely thoughts and feelings arise unbidden and unchosen), but which ones to act on in accordance with one's chosen ethical values.

There is a structural similarity in the emphasis on detachment from specific contingent circumstances, social situations, and personal relationships in both the Enlightenment model of autonomy and the one in contemporary mindfulness. Each has a kind of essential ingredient that renders all such contingencies irrelevant to ethical choice and secures autonomous moral integrity. For Kant, it's reason; for contemporary mindfulness, it's nonjudgmental awareness of the present moment. Again, this is different from more "traditional" forms of Buddhist mindfulness, in which the point is not to nonjudgmentally observe and then act according to one's freely chosen values. Mindfulness in its broadest sense means "remembering," which includes a broader context than just present-moment awareness. It reminds monks of their commitment to a Buddhist way of life, including the often highly specific ethical commitments of monastics (Gethin 2011). Mindfulness is, in this context, a kind of detachment from certain things—those which are forbidden the monastic, those that create unfavorable karma, those that are conducive to hatred, greed, and ignorance—but it includes, as we discussed earlier, a broader mindfulness of the ethical orientation and philosophical worldview of the Buddhist Dharma.

In some articulations, the way modern mindfulness incorporates the ethic of autonomy is that it is seen as creating a kind of interior arena in which moral truths are discovered or self-authenticated, and from which one can then freely act on these discoveries. Present-moment awareness effectively unhooks the thinking, evaluating, judging mind, allowing "objective" interior observation. There is no need, in some accounts, for rigid rules, for the mind will come to understand its own workings, which will naturally lead to acting in ways that avoid one's own and others' suffering. In this sense, this view of meditation has partially absorbed the picture of the Enlightenment's rational autonomous subject in that it presents meditation as opening up an interior domain of relative invulnerability—the Inner Citadel—in which reality within and without is beheld transparently, and this transparency secures right ethical action, freely chosen in accord with the individual's reasoned positions or intuitions—or, in the language of modern mindfulness, "direct experience." Direct experience inoculates the meditator from social conditioning, since this conditioning is an "external" influence contrary to self-determining freedom. It allows the meditator, on this model, to float freely above social and cultural context. This bifurcation of internal and external extends beyond issues of autonomy into well-being. As Michal Pagis points out in her ethnography of Vipassana practitioners in the United States and Israel, there is an "ideology of independence and self-containment" that pervades many meditation communities, the notion that "my happiness is my responsibility" common in popular American culture (2019, 115, 120).

On this model of meditation, one discovers one's own ethical imperatives in the depths of one's mind. Rather than being derived from external rules or social conditioning, they flow forth from within, from the self-authenticating insight of the individual. One version of this might be that detached, empirical observation of one's psychological processes allows for insight into the sources of destructive emotions at the root of unethical behavior, giving one the freedom to choose to act in ethical ways. Another (a more innateist version) is that one discovers one's natural goodness residing deep within—a goodness that is obscured, again, by external factors—which, now unimpeded, flows outward in compassionate action. Lama Govinda, (formerly Luther Hoffman, 1898–1985), illustrates this perspective, as well as the creative braiding together of rationalist, romantic, and Buddhist perspectives of freedom in action:

> Freedom consists in the right application of laws, in making the right use of them, and this depends again on the degree of our knowledge and insight into the nature of things, i.e., into our true nature. To express one's own inner law, one's character, in one's actions, is true self-expression, and self-expression is the hallmark of freedom. (Govinda 1976, 275)

This, what we might call an adjacent "ethic of self-discovery," allows a claim for Buddhism that is easily amalgamated with a modern liberal perspective on morality: "Gotama the Buddha was . . . a real antitraditionalist. He did not offer his teaching as a set of dogmas, but rather as a set of propositions to investigate for him- or herself" (Gunaratana 2002, 34). Ethics are based not on a set of externally imposed regulations but on interior discoveries, again, analogous to the discoveries a scientist makes of the natural world, or on insights into one's unique self that are to be expressed through one's actions in the world.

This dominant conception of the autonomous self, then, is part of a larger, western cultural understanding that now is built-in to our default assumptions and intuitions. Buddhist meditative practices, in their initial introduction to the West, were enlisted into the broad project of acquiring autonomy as conceived along these lines. At the same time, the meditation that was developing in the late twentieth century tended to look askance at political conceptions of freedom, suggesting that the freedom offered by Buddhist meditation practices aimed at a kind of internal invulnerability, while "external" freedom, secured by political activity, was always precarious. In the forward to a book of classical Zen texts, entitled *Zen Essence: The Science of Freedom*, Thomas Cleary writes:

> Zen is the essence of Buddhism, and freedom is the essence of Zen. . . . Yet even while effectively *in* the world, Zen freedom is not essentially *of* the world; it is not the same as a freedom that can be instituted or granted by a social or political system. According to Zen teaching, freedom that depends on things of the world can be undermined, and freedom that can be granted can be taken away. Aiming for freedom that cannot be undermined and cannot be taken away, Zen liberation reaches out from within. By its very nature it cannot enter in from outside the individual mind.
>
> Zen liberation is essentially achieved by special knowledge and perception that penetrate the root of experience. This knowledge and perception free the mind from the arbitrary limitations imposed on it by conditioning, thus awakening dormant capacities of consciousness. . . . Zen cleans the mind for inner perception of its own essential nature; then inner perception of mind's essential purity enables one to remain spontaneously poised and free in all circumstances. (Cleary 1989: 1–2)

Christmas Humphries, a mid-twentieth-century student of Zen, offered a stronger version of this interior invulnerability:

> Learned Audience, what is sitting for meditation? In our School, to sit means to gain absolute freedom and to be mentally unperturbed in all outward circumstances, be they good or otherwise. To meditate means to realise inwardly the imperturbability of the Essence of Mind. (1987, 233)

Such conceptions of Zen, and meditative practices more broadly, were among the many expressions, not just of classical Buddhist ideas, but also of the well-documented late-twentieth-century disillusionment with politics after the failure of the revolutionary movements to produce radical social and political transformation. If the political process could not bring about peace, freedom, and security, perhaps individuals could find these within.

To summarize: this combination of Enlightenment rationalism, romanticism, social psychology, and Orientalism with selected elements of Buddhist doctrine helped generate new individualistic, secularized versions of meditation that aspired to a kind of interior freedom that wove together western liberal conceptions of personal autonomy and ethical agency with Buddhist conceptions of freedom and liberation. It envisioned a kind of interior invulnerability and security, freedom from social norms and external conditioning—an Inner Citadel that at once provided a respite from worldly chaos as well as the conditions for ethical agency.

The Feminist Interrogation of the Autonomous Self

If the Inner Citadel side of secular meditation has absorbed dominant western conceptions of the autonomous subject and its attendant notions of agency, self-transparency, and freedom in the West, it is subject to some of the philosophical and social critiques that have been leveled against them. Indeed, these critiques have been a part of a gradual reappraisal of secular meditation that has given rise to what I am calling the Situated Autonomy model. Many such critiques of ethical agency in terms of the modern concept of the autonomous self have emerged in recent decades, and there is no need to survey them here. The rethinking of these issues in some facets of feminist thought, though, serves as a salient example. Feminist thinkers in recent decades have provided important conceptual resources for investigating and critiquing the inherited idea of the self as a bounded, atomized individual whose ethical imperatives are derived from within. While the classical rational self has often been represented as a generic, ungendered, classless, and raceless individual, feminist theorists have shown how this self is actually coded as male, white, heterosexual, and upper-class. The mind and reason have been traditionally viewed as the male domain, whereas the body and emotion belonged to the female. If, for the Kantian rational subject, emotions and social connections imperil objectivity and therefore impair moral judgment, feminist thinkers have, in contrast, emphasized the socially embedded elements of human experience as necessary for forming ethical judgments. As Ellen Anderson et al. summarize it (in a passage to which I am indebted for the "inner citadel" language):

Prevailing conceptions of the self ignore the multiple, sometimes fractious sources of social identity constituted at the intersections of one's gender, sexual orientation, race, class, age, ethnicity, and so forth. Structural domination and subordination are thought not to penetrate the "inner citadel" of selfhood. Likewise, these conceptions deny the complexity of the dynamic, intrapsychic world of unconscious fantasies, fears, and desires, and they overlook the ways in which such materials intrude upon conscious life. The modern philosophical construct of the rational subject projects a self that is not prey to ambivalence, anxiety, obsession, prejudice, hatred, or violence. A disembodied mind, the body is peripheral—a source of desires for homo economicus to weigh and a distracting temptation for the Kantian ethical subject. . . . Yet, as valuable as rational analysis and free choice undoubtedly are, feminists argue that these capacities do not operate apart from affective, biosocial, socio-economic and other heterogeneous forces that orchestrate the multilayered phenomenon that we call the self. For many feminists, to acknowledge the self's dependency is not to devalue the self but rather to revalue dependency, as well as to call into question the supposed free agency of a self that implicitly corresponds to a masculine ideal. (Anderson, Willett, and Meyers 2020; see also, Meyers 1994)

Some feminist thinkers have gone further in interrogating the autonomous self. Judith Butler, for example, emphasizes the hidden dimensions of subjectivity and ultimately questions whether there is an isolable self at all. The "I," she insists, is not something established by introspection (as Descartes suggested) but only in relation to alterity—what is "not I." It is both a linguistic construction and a constantly shifting relation with the other. She insists that the subject, with its powers of agency, is not something prior to the web of social relations—and, saliently, relations of power—rather, it is through these very relations that the subject is constituted. The paradox is that one is an agent, acting to form oneself as a subject, but also constantly being acted upon by countless other factors that are "not I," and these, inevitably are also a part of the formation of the subject:

I am not only already in the hands of someone else before I start to work with my own hands, but I am also, as it were, in the "hands" of institutions, discourses, environments, including technologies and life processes, handled by an organic and inorganic object field that exceeds the human. In this sense, "I" am nowhere and nothing without the nonhuman. (Butler 2015, 7)

Of course, anyone familiar with Buddhism would find some of these ideas resonant with certain conceptions of nonself and dependent origination, especially in their recent interpretations. Mindfulness entered into the secular imaginary, in part, under the magnetic pull of this notion of the independent, autonomous self as a way of helping secure interior freedom as conceived, in part, by modern, western liberal traditions—again, freedom from internalized societal constraints and freedom to act, think, and feel according to one's own self-generated choices, independent from external circumstances. Yet, certain elements of Buddhism appear, prima facia, to reject some of these tenets and echo these critiques. As we shall see, the fragmentation and decentering of the subject in the late-modern world invite more situated, dependence-oriented interpretations of mindfulness.

Spontaneity and Submission: Alternative Models of Agency in Meditative Traditions

The Dynamics of Agency and Submission

How should we get a foothold on expanded conceptions of ethical autonomy beyond the received notions, and by implication, beyond the Inner Citadel model of meditative practice? Beginning with some anthropological theory and particular cases might help us in a roundabout way. For example, Saba Mahmood's study of modern Islamic groups with very different technologies of the self, and her theoretical interrogation of modern ideas of selfhood and agency, are relevant here. She questions the notion, deeply embedded in the fabric of modern, western liberal notions of autonomy and self-governance, that "human agency primarily consists of acts that challenge social norms and not those that uphold them" (2005: 5). In her study of a conservative Muslim movement, the women's piety movement in Egypt, she details how women enact roles that are antithetical to freedom and agency as conceived in modern secularism. Yet, she insists, a revised conception of agency must make room for how these women, who veil themselves, cultivate virtues of modesty and shyness, and subordinate themselves to males, nevertheless have agency within their cultural context. Freedom, autonomy, and agency are not always and only achieved, she insists, through a desire for freedom from social norms and authority. Rather, a different kind of agency may be achieved through embodying norms and submitting to them until they become deeply embedded in one's habits and ordinary ways of living.

If we transpose Mahmood's analysis to that of Buddhist meditation traditions, we might find that bringing western liberal assumptions about agency to them may obscure how meditation works for at least some practitioners. Lina Verchery does just this in her study of Buddhist nuns at the Avatamsaka Sagely Monastery in Alberta, Canada, a part of the Dharma Realm Buddhist Association founded by Master Xuan Hua (Verchery 2015). Nuns at the monastery have a rigorous schedule, rising at 3:30 AM, eating just one meal a day, keeping constantly busy, living by strict rules of the Vinaya monastic code, and having neither privacy nor possessions. Meditation in this context is just one aspect of "cultivation" (*xiu xing*, 修行), a term frequently used in Dharma Realm circles, which includes the development of ethical virtues, states of mind, dispositions, and wisdom. By subjecting themselves to the rigors of monastic life and submitting to its many rules, norms, and disciplines, the nuns cultivate virtues and characteristics valued in their tradition and thus strive to live their chosen ethics. Meditation is a part of this cultivation, but it is embedded in a larger way of life subject to authority and hierarchy, which are seen as necessary to producing the kinds of persons they want to become. They experience, according to Verchery, a sense of freedom and ease in not having to concern themselves with money or possessions or other worldly matters. The life of the nuns is also very much one of community and collective endeavor rather than an individual one. Each individual sees herself as a model for laypeople of dedication to the Dharma but also as a check on the other nuns, encouraging them in their own self-cultivation and helping them to conform to the demanding monastic life.[3]

We can infer that the insights gained in their meditation are not simply freeform, self-directed, and self-authenticated but rather are shaped and nurtured by close study of scripture and consultation with their teachers. Such a rulebound life, in which individual autonomy appears minimized, adherence to rules emphasized, and responsibility to others—fellow monastics, as well as laity—is valued over independent autonomy might hardly be recognized as a pursuit of freedom in a modern, liberal sense.

Trained Spontaneity and Ritual in Zen

Zen monastic life in Japan offers another example of a contemplative tradition that complicates the standard modern picture of agency, autonomy, and spontaneity, and their relation to meditative practice. As Shulman has pointed out regarding early texts like the *Sutta on the Foundations of Mindfulness*, the hope is that the reconfiguration of subjectivity toward, for example, calm, detachment, and compassion, away from greed, hatred, and agitation will become naturalized and part of one's enduring dispositions, no longer requiring overt thought and effort (Shulman 2010). Activities that manifest valued dispositions then become spontaneous. The value of this spontaneity, little discussed in Indian Buddhism, became more explicit in East Asian Buddhism as it took on board ideas originating in Confucian and Daoist traditions.

As we have discussed, in some Zen literature, spontaneity could look unruly, iconoclastic, and antinomian. In the classical anecdotes, Zen masters appear to flout convention and common morality, even Buddhist morality. They seemed to value dramatic, spontaneous action over doctrinally correct words—smacking students or kicking over a water jar in response to a question, cutting a cat in two in response to the failure to answer a question. Such stories of iconoclastic freedom appealed immensely to postromantic, countercultural fans of Zen in the twentieth century but are belied by even a cursory introduction to life in a Zen training monastery. The picture of agency we get there is much more like that of the monastics at the Avatamsaka Sagely Monastery mentioned above. All activities are ritualized, formulaic, and thoroughly rule-bound, from getting out of bed to going to the bathroom to eating to chanting to meditating. The *dokusan* room, where students have private meetings with their masters to display their understanding, is reputed to be an arena in which anything can happen, and students who can show their spontaneous understanding are likely to impress the master more than ones who are faking it or just being impulsive. Yet, for the most part, Zen monastic life is as regimented as a military unit. Great effort is required in monastics' training to inhabit formal, ritualized monastic comportment and subdue the interpretations, bodily movements, dispositions, and habitual thought and feeling that they inhabited before training. When monastics completely embody this new way of being in the world, when it becomes naturalized, then they are thought to be enacting their buddha nature spontaneously. Ritualized activity is designed to help the student cultivate very specific ways of thinking, feeling, and being—those of a fully awakened buddha, which the student, ironically, already is. The term *gyōji* encompasses this sense of "sustained practice" in which one brings the same sense of ritual comportment to everyday activities that they do to ceremonial activities (Borup 2008). Monks often recite verses that provide sacralized interpretations of every phenomenon and activity—eating, sweeping, using the bathroom. This is, however, not considered an instrumental process, since, the tradition insists, one is already awakened. So, *zazen* and the other ritualized practices are expressions of one's already-awakened nature, which is said to be present even if one has no awareness of it. In this sense, they are "enactment rituals"—you act like the buddha you already are (Leighton 2007). Especially in the Sōtō school of Zen, whether you *feel* like a buddha is less important than embodying the activities and comportment of a buddha. Other East Asian Buddhist traditions have analogous understandings of ritual. For example, Shingon rituals for identifying the body, mind, and speech with that of a buddha are procedures "viewed as an enactment of buddhahood" in which "the practitioner literally mimics the body, speech, and mind of the Tathāgatha" (Sharf 2001, 196). The mimetic enactment of how the tradition imagines a buddha would act does not seem like freedom and spontaneity on the modern western model, yet it is one of the ways that Buddhist traditions themselves have conceived of freedom.

Apparent antiritualistic eruptions of spontaneity, however, are included in Zen training, illustrating a tension between highly regulated modes of life and the occasional sudden rupture of routine. Such disruptions, however, are also a part of the tradition rather than a departure from it. Dale Wright illustrates this tension with reference to a scene in the Korean movie, *Mandala*, in which, in response to a *kōan* presented by the Zen master during a formal, ritualized lecture (*teishō*), a monk jumps up and grabs the master's stick and breaks it. In the modern, post-Suzuki interpretation of Zen, this would seem to represent the triumph of the autonomous, spontaneous self against the dry, empty authority and formalism of the institution—the very essence of Zen (as well as, coincidentally, modern liberalism). And yet, as Wright points out, "even this outrageous anti-ritual gesture is encompassed by the ritual occasion as a whole. Although perhaps shocked by the audacity of the young monk, all in attendance understand how defiance of ritual is almost as traditional a gesture in Zen as the ritual itself—an 'anti-ritual ritual'—that had been modeled for them in the classic texts of Zen" (Wright 2007, 5). The fact that pervasive ritual decorum might include some moments of apparent rupture from the regimented comportment expected of a monk illustrates the sophisticated understanding that the tradition itself has of the dynamics of structure and antistructure, of the tension between deeply inhabiting a prescribed way of being and the inability for mere conformity to an ideal to adequately encapsulate the pursuit of an awakened life.

The Zen monastic example offers another way to conceive of meditative life conferring disciplined agency within a context that is not so much focused on the decontextualized free will of the individual self but rather on the mastery of certain ritual forms and ethical dispositions that shape character. Although this way might make room for strategic inversions of the traditional structures of authority, as well as ruptures in ritual behavior and prescribed comportment, freedom and spontaneity here are not primarily the transcendence or contravention of social norms and the carrying out of one's sovereign, independent will but rather the ability to inhabit a particular form of life with complete "naturalness" and grace. Such ideas of agency and spontaneity are deeply embedded in East Asian thought and go back to early Daoist and Confucian conceptions of "effortless action" (*wuwei*) that worked their way into East Asian forms of Buddhism.

Meditation and Autonomy

The examples of the Avatamsaka Sagely Monastery and of Zen monasteries in Japan alert us to ways in which the relationship between meditation, agency, and ethics may be configured other than on a purely binary model of the autonomous individual's assertion of self-directed agency against the norms of community and the demands of society, tradition, social conditioning, or other "external" influences. Instead, there is a more complex and contextual embracing of certain norms rather than others, acting on certain values rather than others, cultivation of particular skills and sensibilities, submission to certain influences and resistance to others. There is another, converse, implication. The person who conceives herself free of all social constraints, answerable only to the authentic imperatives of her individual conscience, is also inevitably acting within certain prescribed forms of rebellion and authenticity that also have their own protocol, like the monk who grabs the master's stick or the punk with immaculately spiked hair.

How does the ethic of autonomy and the enhancement of moral agency through meditative practices look through the lens of these examples, then? Mahmood characterizes moral agency "(a) in terms of the capacities and skills required to undertake particular kinds of moral actions; and (b) as ineluctably bound up with the historically and culturally specific disciplines through which a subject is formed. The paradox of subjectivation [is] that the capacity for action is enabled and created by specific relations of subordination" (2005, 29). She offers as an example a pianist who submits herself to the authority of a teacher, the rigors of regular practice, and the tradition of a particular musical style—something that requires the abnegation of agency in one sense, but is required for the acquisition of agency in another sense: her capacity to master her instrument. Likewise, the training of meditators, while it may require the submission to discipline and the curbing of desires, enables meditators to create the kind of "selves" that they strive to cultivate. The training of the monastery (and even, in a less urgent way, the training of the secular mindfulness class) shapes and hones particular sensibilities and moral capacities rather than simply clearing away socially constructed impositions on the pure capacity to see things as they are and act according to one's sovereign will. Freedom in this sense is, in Maggie Nelson's words, "knotted up with so-called unfreedom, producing marbled experiences of compulsion, discipline, possi-bility, and surrender" (Nelson 2021, 9).

So, how does this relate to specifically secular forms of contemporary medi-tation? The fact that such practices have now spread not only beyond the mon-astery, but beyond Buddhism itself, means that they are applied to a dizzying array of purposes as diverse as work, romantic relationships, dying, political engagement, health, and sports. They have found their way into countless niches of modern life and are applied not only to "this-worldly" purposes in general but to *this* job, *this* marriage, *this* illness, *this* tennis game, *this* social problem. Some of these applications might well cultivate enhanced autonomy within a particular set of norms, whether of the dominant social imaginary or of a narrower subculture that resists those norms. A practitioner might use meditation to cultivate the courage to go against the gender roles of her com-munity in order to pursue a particular career; another might use mindfulness to make himself more focused and productive at work, cultivating capacities rewarded by dominant cultural expectations.

For socially and culturally embedded beings, autonomy is situated within particular contexts and comes up against specific barriers. If we conceive of the emancipatory potentials of meditative practices as simply liberating practitioners from all social conditioning and habituated patterns of thought, feeling, and desire into a space of utterly unfettered freedom of self-generated activity, we miss much of how meditation works on the ground. These practices recondition and retrain thoughts and feelings in certain directions rather than others, carving out spaces for practitioners to inhabit distinc-tive ways of being in the world that are created and maintained socially. They foster the embodiment of certain norms and dispositions while at the same time curtailing, attenuating, and challenging others. Mindfulness does, as is often claimed, allow practitioners to more clearly see their habitual patterns and their limitations, but it also—implicitly or explicitly—comes packaged with suggestions for alternative patterns. Such practices are conducive to a freedom that is nuanced and complex, shaped by particular contexts the prac-titioner inhabits.

Even a casual meditation practice in a secular setting suggests certain dis-ciplines, values, and norms as part of the package. The difference that the contemporary contexts make is that these values and norms may vary wildly, from those of corporate culture to New Age self-care to antiracist activism to horseback riding. It is not only nuns in the highly controlled disciplinary context of the monastery who practice their meditation in a situated dialectic of agency and subordination. Ordinary lay practitioners, including the most secularized of meditators, do too. In a multitude of ways, meditators derive their insights, moral vision, bodily comportment, and affective habits not merely from a private realm but from the various cultures and subcultures with which they are in continuing, constitutive relationships. In contrast to the Inner Citadel model, which tends to conceive of the benefits of meditation as limited to interior states of mind and is skeptical of "political" applications of meditation, the Situated Autonomy orientation has allowed meditators to expand the deployments of the practice to a wide array of activities, personal, social, and political.

The Situated Autonomy model makes more sense of how meditation actually works in lives embedded in particular, contingent contexts. It coheres more with current understandings in anthropology, sociology, religious studies, philosophy, psychology, and cognitive science than does the Inner Citadel model. How, then, do we envision the way meditation might enhance situated autonomy? I'll continue this line of questioning from another angle in the next chapter, offering a theoretical account of how we might see this enhanced sense of autonomy in terms of the concept of affordances. I will also discuss some of the recent novel applications of meditation to particular social and political movements, applications that had not really emerged earlier when the Inner Citadel orientation was dominant.

11

Affordances, Disruption, and Activism

Navigating the Internal Affordance Landscape

Many people report having profound experiences of inner freedom during meditation. These experiences give them new perspectives on things, provide insights into their own psychological processes, and bring forth a sense of greater autonomy in the world. They might feel transported beyond the mundane, beyond concern for how others think of them, beyond their social roles, their tensions with others, their fears of wither and decay. They may feel like they have touched something beyond the physical world or beyond ordinary thought and feeling. But presumably they all come back eventually to the mundane world and must deal with the quotidian realities of life anew: how to navigate work, relationships, parenting. Meditative practices may propel practitioners out of their ordinary world, but can also be a means of managing the intricacies of that world. As one popular title puts it: *After the Ecstasy, the Laundry* (Kornfield 2000).

Big, transcendent, life-changing contemplative experiences are by nature difficult to pin down and are, perhaps, better expressed in poetry or autobiography than in theoretical analysis (though Buddhist philosophy has a long tradition of such analysis). We can nevertheless delve into the more modest, earthy phenomenology of what happens in the typical, everyday experiences of meditation, particularly with regard to our inquiry into freedom and ethical agency. I'll refrain from speculating here on the far reaches of freedom and liberation that meditation might afford the advanced practitioner and consider, instead, the more everyday kinds of heightened agency that meditation might help cultivate.[1] In this chapter, I want to begin thinking through this issue in two ways. First, I consider how we might conceive of the meditative practices we have been examining as providing a way of making explicit what is implicit, half-conscious, and part of individuals' default ways of being in the world. This sets up a dynamic of pursuing and subduing "affordances," potentials for activity, be they physical or psychological. Analyzing meditative practices in terms of affordances offers an alternative to the Theater of the Mind model of mental activity, discussed in chapter 2. Second, I touch on how

Rethinking Meditation. David L. McMahan, Oxford University Press. © Oxford University Press 2023.
DOI: 10.1093/oso/9780197661741.003.0011

the ethical dimensions of contemporary forms of meditation have recently been extended beyond the search for interior liberation and brought to bear on external barriers to autonomy, such as oppressive social structures or environmental threats. This movement to bring meditation to social and political transformation, while an extension of the underlying logic of meditation in the secular imaginary, signals a significant shift in thinking about what how meditation works and the work meditation does.

Physical, Cultural, and Ethical Affordances

The concept of affordances began in ecological psychology and has spread into several different fields, including cross-cultural psychology, cognitive science, and design. The original idea, developed by James Gibson in his 1966 book, *The Senses Considered as Perceptual Systems*, is that affordances are features of things in the environment that offer (afford) organisms cues as to how they might interact with these things. That is, they are particular opportunities and possibilities a thing provides for behavior. A tree might afford a person or a squirrel climbing. A door handle affords grasping and turning. "The affordances of the environment are what it offers the animal, what it provides or furnishes, either for good or ill" (Gibson 1979, 127).

On this model, we do not simply experience the world as a passive subject perceiving and interpreting representations of neutral objects; rather, we encounter it as a complex array of possibilities for action or opportunities for behavior. According to some theorists, affordances present themselves without need of explicit representation. One reaches for a door handle without explicitly thinking about how it works or making a conscious decision about how to turn it. Moreover, different affordances will present themselves depending on the purposes and activities of the perceiver. A chair affords sitting for a weary walker but it might also serve to block the door against an intruder. While most theories of affordances see them as objective properties of the environment that might be exploitable by an animal, I am inclined (perhaps influenced by my study of Buddhist thought) to see them as neither objective properties nor subjective projections but as relations. As Anthony Chemero puts it: "[affordances are] relations between particular aspects of animals and particular aspects of situations" (Chemero 2009, 139). The concept of affordances departs from a representational concept of the relationship of subject and object, revealing ways to think about this relationship as more intertwined, with subjects shaped by, attuned to, and interrelated with things in the world in intimate, constitutive ways.

In recent decades the idea of affordances has stretched considerably, bending it closer in relevance to our subjects of meditation, culture, ethics, and agency. Some theorists have expanded the concept to include "cultural affordances," which include "possibilities for action, the engagement with which depends on agents' skillfully leveraging explicit or implicit expectations, norms, conventions, and cooperative social practices in their ability to correctly infer (implicitly or explicitly) the culturally specific sets of expectations of which they are immersed. These are expectations about how to interpret other agents, and the symbolically and linguistically mediated social world" (Ramstead et al. 2016). Further expanding the concept into the domain of ethical agency, Webb Keane offers the idea of "ethical affordances," first suggesting that an affordance is "not just a physical object but *anything at all* that people can experience, such as emotions, bodily movements, habitual practices, linguistic forms, laws, etiquette, or narratives, [which possess] an indefinite number of combinations of properties" (Keane 2015, 30; italics original). Within this broad set of phenomena, ethical affordances, then, are "the opportunities that any experiences might offer as people evaluate themselves, other persons, and their circumstances" (31).

Such a capacious view of affordances, while it may stretch the concept considerably, allows us to extend it to practices of the self by which people reflexively engage in observing and shaping their own thoughts, emotions, and interpretations of things. Reflexive practices like meditation take as the object of attention not some feature of the environment but one's own internal features, (which, as we have insisted before, are not just phenomena "inside the head" but are always organically and systemically connected to the environment, to others, and to culture). Such practices call forth an "internal affordance landscape" (Metzinger 2017). The affordances evoked in this case provide various opportunities not just for physical action but also for "mental action" (McClelland, 2020) including focusing attention, disciplining emotions, redirecting thought to particular subjects, and reinterpreting situations along the lines of particular moral, philosophical, or religious views.

Reflexive and Meditative Affordances

Thinking of meditative practices as providing opportunities to put a variety of affordances into play while resisting or rejecting other affordances allows us to think with more precision about the Situated Autonomy model of meditation. On this interpretation, autonomy contains a dynamic tension between denial, affirmation, and reinterpretation of certain features of the internal affordance landscape brought into greater focus by reflexive, introspective practices. Such practices create a sense of greater autonomy in that they bring about a level of heightened, thematic awareness, inducing explicit consciousness of what is normally implicit, and offering expanded opportunities to refuse, pursue, and reinterpret certain affordances according to a particular ethical vision.

Returning to the example of mindful eating offers an example of these dynamics and how they might work in different cultural contexts with disparate repertoires of cultural affordances. In the context of the Vinaya, the rules for Buddhist monastics, we've seen in chapter 4 that mindful eating has to do with curbing the appetites and detachment from the physical allure of food, as well as the physical comportment and decorum expected of a monk. Two values are built in to this practice: first, the value of renunciation of worldly pleasures, which amounts to a judgment on their relative uselessness and the danger that attachment to them will hinder progress toward awakening. Second is the expectation that the monk should display this detachment from worldly pleasures to others in order to inspire them and demonstrate dedication to the Dharma. An ethic of renunciation is fundamental to mindful eating in the Vinaya. Mindfulness in this situation disrupts the implicit affordance offered by food that might induce one to simply grab and eat as much as one wants and in whatever manner. This disruption allows eating to become a matter of explicit awareness so that the many rules about eating—an alternative array of affordances—can be actualized. The food still affords eating, but mindfulness requires remaining attentive to the particular ways a monk is expected to eat. Of course, all eating involves the learning of an intricate grammar of ingestion—manners that we all learn as children. The Vinaya illustrates the challenges of learning a new and even more intricate grammar for monastics, which they must usually learn as adults.

Mindful eating in the context of secular meditative practices also disrupts the habitual affordances offered by a meal, but the values brought to meal are different. They might be conveyed in the sentiment, often expressed in contemporary Dharma literature, that we are always so busy and distracted that we are not fully living our lives but instead go through the motions of eating, walking, working, and playing half-consciously. "Sleepwalking through life," is a common phrase in this literature. As an antidote, mindful eating brings about a heightened appreciation (again) of the subtleties and nuances of eating and thus allows for a richer experience. This does not imply a purely hedonistic approach; in fact, mindful eating is often employed today as a technique for imposing discipline, such as that required for maintaining a healthy weight. The tacitly, prereflectively apprehended affordances offered by a meal (again, conditioned by one's childhood training in manners, which have become habituated, thus prereflective) are disrupted by a mindful attention that rejects certain values and embraces others—in this case, the rejection of constant busyness, distraction, and inattention pervasive in contemporary life, and embracing the value of slowing down and appreciating one's present-moment experience and, therefore, living one's life fully. The world-affirming ethic of appreciation generates certain affordances that are made available by training and reinterpreting the experience of eating within a particular culture of mindfulness. Practitioners are taught to seek out and value particular experiences—for example, noting the subtle flavors and textures of one's food—and to avoid and devalue others—stuffing oneself while watching television. Even "nonjudgmental awareness" cannot escape such evaluation: one must learn to discern when one is successfully pulling off "living fully in the moment" or appreciating one's life—or one's dinner.

Mindfulness grants heightened reflexive illumination of impulses that might usually be only semiconscious (the impulse to grab as much food as possible, fill one's mouth greedily, etc.) and then subjects them to evaluation according to one's training. Successful application of mindfulness necessitates a commitment to the ethical value in play—renouncing worldly pleasures for the monastic or appreciating life fully for the practitioner of contemporary mindfulness. Similar analyses could apply to a variety of ethically relevant affordances, like the acquiring of possessions, sexual opportunities, and speaking to others. Even when framed as nonjudgmental awareness, mindfulness is always value-laden, bending activity to certain possibilities rather than others.

Interpretive Affordances

One particular feature of the internal affordance landscape that meditative practices address is what we might think of as "interpretive affordances," opportunities to interpret phenomena in certain ways. These can involve highly contextual circumstances—subtle affordances that invite particular interpretations: "this situation is hopeless" versus "this situation is manageable," or "this person enrages me" versus "I am aware of my rage, observing it, and not getting carried away by it." In classical traditions of Buddhist meditation, we've seen how bodies could be interpreted (or, according to the tradition, misinterpreted) as stable, desirable, and beautiful. This construal is disrupted by meditations on the body that offer alternative interpretive affordances suggesting its fragility, foulness, and finitude.

Some Buddhist meditations contain ontological assertions affording radical reinterpretations of reality in the broadest sense. Consider this brief meditation instruction from the Tibetan teacher and scholar from the Nyingma school, Chögyal Terdag Lingpa (1646–1714):

> The alternation of thoughts of happiness and suffering, desire and aversion, is nothing more than the play of luminous emptiness and mind. Without altering whatever arises, look at its nature, and you will perceive it as great bliss. (quoted in Ricard 2013, ch. 1 [ebook])

This quotation sets up a particular nexus of interpretive affordances. It invites the reader to reflexively attend to present-moment internal phenomena and to take a certain stance on each moment of "happiness and suffering, desire and aversion" as, in reality, quite different from how they are actually apprehended. The quotation, therefore, suggests a refusal of the habitual interpretive affordances—ways of interpreting one's experience—based on the ontological assertion that these interpretations are rooted in a faulty understanding of reality. This would include, for example, attributing one's happiness or sadness to contingent circumstances—I lost my job, therefore I am sad; I am eating a delicious pear, therefore I am happy. Then comes the offering of an alternative set of interpretive affordances: all such experiences are to be reinterpreted as mere fluctuations of consciousness, like ripples on a lake. Watching them without altering them eventually leads to the realization that these fluctuations are actually the "play of luminous emptiness and mind." Observing the thoughts without altering them, combined with the seemingly contrary effort to apprehend them as luminous, is combined with a further interpretive affordance: reinterpreting all of one's experiences as "great bliss."

Here we come to a tension within the instructions themselves. The passage suggests that in order to achieve this realization of "great bliss" one merely has to leave thoughts alone and let the mind settle into its "natural state"—a calm, luminous awareness. We could read this as the pacifying of all perceptions of affordances. And yet, at least the initial attempts at such a practice are inevitably complex, involving imagination, aspiration, and struggle to affirm certain interpretations and reject others. They involve keeping concentrated on each passing moment, refusing the affordances of a particular interpretation of the experience of these moments, and being pulled forward by the promise of a radical transformation in how the constant fluctuations of mind are perceived—"great bliss." The quotation is not simply an ontological statement of doctrine but an invitation to labor to experience the world and one's mind in a particular, counterintuitive way.

Many strands of Tibetan meditation quite consciously make use of this capacity to restructure the practitioner's subjectivity through the imagination, for example, Tantric visualizations in which one imagines oneself as a buddha or bodhisattva. But even the practice we are discussing, which would seem in some ways to be the opposite—that is, aiming at the quieting of all imagination—must, at least at first, employ imagination, interpretation, and restructuring of the internal affordance landscape. Some meditative traditions might insist, if pushed to adopt our terminology, that *all* affordances must be refused and one must stop chasing any interpretation whatsoever in order to arrive at the mind's "natural state." Even here, however, at least the initial efforts must involve navigating a complex array of interpretive affordances in the difficult attempt to reimagine the significance of the texture of one's very life as something very different from how it initially appears.

The dialectical refusal and embracing of interpretive affordances would seem to be a part of many, if not all, Buddhist meditative practices. They are most stark in the innateist traditions, which insist that each individual is, in reality, already an awakened being with all of the qualities of a buddha. Zen texts, for example, insist that the world and ourselves are actually quite different from how we typically perceive and understand them. Rather than isolated individuals and objects, everything is "one mind." Rather than being a finite, bumbling, limited individual, one is really a fully awakened buddha. Thus, one must arouse "great doubt" in all ordinary thoughts and perceptions, "great faith" in the possibility of coming to understand how things really are, and "great determination" to achieve this understanding. One must suspend one's habitual interpretive affordances, imagine others that are not yet actualized, and strive to realign one's lived experience with the not-yet-actualized. This entails a radical dereification of the entirety of one's affordance landscape in favor of one that is only present in the imagination (at least initially).

In more constructivist meditative practices as well, practitioners are told that their ordinary experience yields a faulty apprehension of the world and that meditative inquiry can remedy this delusion. In Pali accounts, one mistakes oneself for a singular, isolated "self," when in actuality one is constituted by five different, intertwined processes, the aggregates (*skandhas*). At a still deeper level of analysis, one is the constant flow of momentary, interdependent *dharmas* conditioned by past karma. And in contemporary secular contexts, other constellations of interpretive affordances are offered. For example, in mindfulness-based cognitive therapy, one's "thoughts" are held in ontological suspicion. Practitioners are invited to dereify them, interpreting them as "just thoughts"—"don't believe everything you think!" They are reconceived as unreal, and thus the affordances they offer—whether they are interpretations of others' behavior, self-images, judgments about others or oneself—are neutralized, or at least their power is temporarily attenuated.

These examples help illuminate the processes by which meditative practices might heighten a sense of agency by enhancing reflexive aware-ness of affordances available at a prereflective level, disrupting the compul-sive momentum toward acting on them, and opening up different affordances embedded in alternative values, ideas, and interpretations presented at a more conscious level of attention. Perhaps the transformative potentials in this interplay of affordances are more radical in practices that explicitly in-vite practitioners to question the very reality of all perceived phenomena. Meditative practices in this sense offer the possibility to deeply reinterpret and restructure ontological assumptions and potentials for activity, whether this is ethically relevant activity in the world or the activity of interpreting how the world really is. This approach also suggests how such practices offer these possibilities not in some abstract way involving the properties of ra-tional selves but as part of the flow of subjectivity embedded in particular contexts—an increased freedom *not* to do what one is habituated to do, as well as the freedom to clarify and enact different interpretations, evaluations, judgments, and courses of action. This might include, for example, freedom not to dive headlong into rage, not to interpret a situation with all-consuming fear, not to impulsively say something harmful. Such increased freedom is not like the autonomy of the Kantian subject, floating freely above contin-gent circumstances, making abstract, rational moral evaluations, resisting the contaminating influence of society. Rather it involves an assemblage of embodied, cognitive, and affective skills functioning together in particular sit-uated contexts. It entails reflexive observation of impulses and emotions that might ordinarily remain preconscious, and the deployment of skills of scru-tiny, judgment, interpretation, and evaluation (Am I really appreciating my food right now? Stop daydreaming and focus! Is this a hint of "great bliss"?). Like learning a new language, such a process requires being embedded in a context, a social imaginary, with a repertoire of available values, concepts, and markers of progress. Thus it involves not just an *internal* affordance land-scape but the various cultural and ethical affordances offered by traditions, be they the rich, orthodox versions of Buddhism or the more recent "traditions" of health, well-being, or personal growth in contemporary secular/spiritual contexts.

I realize that talk of such "internal" affordances may rub some the wrong way. After all, the idea was developed to overcome the Theater of the Mind view, in which the bifurcation of everything into internal or external is too stark. But the point here is to offer a view of meditative practices that is not like a pair of eyes looking into a dark room at what was always there. Instead it emphasizes the fact that the mind is enactive; rather than passively perceiving representations, it actively seeks and probes both the "internal" and "external," for different possibilities of action, whether that action is physical, social, or reflexive. Mindfulness in this respect slows down this process so that, rather than being impulsively drawn forward by affordances (whether those of food, compulsive internal dialogue, or sudden rage at another person), one can manage agency in a more calm and capacious way, which increases one's array of possible activities, attitudes, intentions, and interpretations.

Ruptures, Breakdown, and Ethics

In the account I have given so far, part of what is going on is the reconfiguring of the affordance landscape—setting up and nurturing reflexive, ethical, and interpretive affordances according to a tradition of meditative practice and letting other affordances wither, thus gradually transforming the practitioner's way of being in the world. We have examined ways of thinking about medita- tion as a means of enhancing situated autonomy and providing a way of nav- igating away from a set of cultural, interpretive, and ethical affordances built in to one's default social imaginary and navigating toward affordances in an alternative one. But at this point, we might ask whether this interpretation suggests that meditation simply navigates practitioners to another social im- aginary in which one is then similarly enmeshed—or to put it more bluntly, trapped—be it a rigorous tradition like that of the nuns at the Avatamsaka Sagely Monastery or the less robust imaginaries of contemporary secular health and well-being. Is this sense of enhanced autonomy, in other words, just exchanging one set of cultural constraints for another? Here I want to address further how we might think about the process of disruption—of the rupture from the habitual, default modes of thinking and feeling that medita- tion might provide—and its implications for new ways in which meditation is currently being thought of as a means not only of personal liberation but also of social change.

We have been focusing on the role of meditation in building new dispositions, interpretations, propensities toward ethical action, as well as ways of physical comportment within a particular social context. As I suggested in chapter 4, this is similar to the construction of something like what the sociologist Pierre Bourdieu called a *habitus*, a set of durable dispositions and bodily comport- ment that is learned but becomes thoroughly naturalized and habitual. For Bourdieu, this process involves the largely unconscious "practical mimesis"

that inculcates the habits, values, taste, and comportment of a particular social class (1980: 73). In some respects, the example of Zen monastic training
would seem to fit this model; however, Bourdieu's insistence that acquiring a
habitus is a process of the norms of a particular culture or subculture seeping
into a person's character through preconscious imitation is inadequate to our
cases. In contrast to these largely unconscious social mechanisms, meditative
practices bring explicit awareness to the movements of body, breath, thought,
and feeling. They help to train practitioners in both subtle, half-conscious
ways (through, for instance, the emulation of a teacher and her behavior) and
in more conscious ways (through explicit teaching of morality, what to look
for and value in experience, how to imagine the world and one's relationship
to it, how to "act" like an awakened being). The acquiring of a *habitus* through
meditation, therefore, involves the conscious, often arduous, creation of durable dispositions not only through conscious training in establishing them
but also through a critique, or in some cases a dereification or dismantling
of one's former *habitus*, or at least elements of it. For Bourdieu, the *habitus*
is something in which one is in some measure trapped because it is largely
constructed of unconscious habits and dispositions and not a matter of conscious reflexive consideration. It is nonnegotiable because it is outside of explicit thought from the beginning. A meditation practice, however, attempts
to excavate those habits and dispositions, expose them to conscious reflection, and transform or transcend them, thereby establishing alternative ways
of being.

How might we conceive of the dialectical process of the deconstruction and
reconstruction of a *habitus* (or parts of it) through meditative practice? The
anthropologist Jarrett Zigon makes a distinction between ethics and morality
that might be salient if extended to meditation. "Morality," he contends, has
to do with our ordinary, unreflective being-in-the-world, where we habitually take up the moral dispositions of everyday life that are taken for granted
in a shared cultural context. "Ethics," in contrast, emerges at a moment of
"breakdown," when there is a dilemma, temptation, disagreement, or novel
situation that one's ordinary, unquestioned, and unreflective mode of being
cannot adequately address. One is forced to "step-away [sic] and figure out,
work through and deal with the situation-at-hand" (Zigon 2007, 137). Such
a "stepping-away" thematizes the problem explicitly, extracting it from the
normal flow of unreflective life. "For the very process of stepping-out and
responding to the breakdown in various ways alters, even if ever so slightly,
the aspect of being-in-the-world that is the unreflective moral dispositions.
It is in the moment of breakdown, then, that it can be said that people work

on themselves, and in so doing, alter their very way of being-in-the-world" (138). The breakdown is similar to what Foucault called "problematization" or "thought," which "allows one to step back from this way of acting or reacting [the taken-for-granted], to present it to oneself as an object of thought and to question it as to its meaning, its conditions, and its goals. Thought is freedom in relation to what one does, the motion by which one detaches oneself from it, establishes it as an object, and reflects on it as a problem" (Foucault 2000, 117, cited in Zigon 2007, 137).

Some meditative practices at once cultivate a "breakdown" of the taken-for-granted, a dereification of default assumptions and habituated dispositions, and also provide alternatives to restabilize and reconceive things in different ways. They may also push a practitioner toward a crisis of ethical action by dismantling the usual categories, values, and dispositions through which one navigates moral activity in the world. The contexts in which meditation occurs, however, always supply, implicitly or explicitly, alternative categories, values, and dispositions from a different imaginary, whether from a particular school of Buddhism or a more secularized culture of meditation. These alternatives may, themselves, be more ethically demanding than the default, everyday mode of the dominant social imaginary, or they may ultimately encourage acquiescence to it—a return to home after an invigorating break. It all depends on factors surrounding meditation, the context in which meditation is embedded and which supplies the alternative to the default imaginary.

Some might object to assimilating meditative reflexivity to a moment of "problematization" or "thought," given contemporary meditation's view of "thoughts" and "figuring out" as antithetical to true meditation. Meditation, this view insists, simply allows thoughts to arise and passively observes them, something that seems less engaged and goal-directed than actively working out an ethical problem. The very focus on the present moment cuts off deliberation, planning, and conceptualization and thus frees the mind from these processes of moral reflection. Yet, even in that more detached mode of observation, space is created that can allow for an expanded accounting of the available possibilities for acting and interpreting—an expansion of the internal affordance landscape. In the stepping back from the constant pursuit of habituated affordances, aspects of the lived world appear more explicit and delineated than if one were simply absorbed in everyday, default intuitions and activities. Thus, even if the practice in question is a kind of minimal "bare observation," the practitioner is nevertheless doing work toward clarifying, evaluating, imagining, and interpreting, guided by some underlying moral vision.

Meditation, Social Change, and "Interruptive Agency"

In meditation practices in which the practitioner reflexively observes "what comes up," space is created to inventory possible ethical affordances and act consciously from a considered ethical standpoint instead of being propelled by the unreflective, everyday impulses shaped by the practitioner's dominant social imaginary. This does not mean one has broken free of all external social constraints, as more romantic interpretations of meditation suggest, or that one is a disengaged, autonomous, rational subject invulnerable to social and material conditions. One is always embedded in a social context and limited by certain possibilities therein. And yet, the reflexive moment that meditation can provide may foster the expansion of those possibilities, stimulating novel interpretations and imaginings not possible if one were simply being swept along unreflectively immersed in the momentum one's native *habitus*. The heightened reflexivity fostered in these practices, along with the dereifying elements inherent in them, may increase the fluidity of the moral imagination, foster breaking free from calcified habits of thought and valuation, and nurture new combinations of elements in a culturally available repertoire, allowing novel interpretations and actions to emerge and agency to extend beyond dominant ideological structures.

Such experiences can obviously be deeply meaningful and rewarding on a personal level. But of how much value is this sense of internal freedom and the possibilities of self-transformation if you are a woman in a deeply misogynist society, a minority in a racist culture, a citizen in an authoritarian regime, or a resident of an island nation about to be submerged in rising seas? The answer is almost certainly not "none"; nevertheless, some meditators have responded to such questions by attempting to extend the work that meditation does beyond personal experience to ethical agency as a social and political actor. The disruptive aspect of meditation—creating space for ruptures from default modes of thinking—has invited, in ways unique to this historical moment, the question of how meditation might be brought to bear on social and political issues. The way thinkers have recently thought about this issue provides us with another way to reflect on the question of agency and freedom in relation to meditative practices.

Political theorist Shannon Mariotti, for example, considers the potentialities for meditation to interrupt default modes of thought in service of democratic reform through a kind of "interruptive agency." Drawing from thinkers like Eve Sedgwick, Michel de Certeau, and Jacques Rancière, she suggests that:

Practices of meditation and mindfulness are . . . spaces and places where users can and do employ tactics that reclaim the authority of their own experience, where they enact forms of interruptive agency that disrupt constraining and containing systems. Zen practice can help unsettle the default modes of perception built into us by modernity in ways that can generate creative and imaginative impulses that allow us to enact other ways of being in the world. (2020, 489)

Mariotti argues, for example, that meditative practice can be employed in disrupting internalized structures of systemic racism.[2] Another example of this rupture of the ordinary that presents new possibilities is the potential for meditation to reclaim the "attentional commons." This is an idea pioneered by Matthew Crawford, who suggests that attention should be treated as a valuable resource that we hold in common, like water or air, that is increasingly dominated by advertising and corporate messaging (Crawford 2015). Meditation, for Mariotti, is a way to "reclaim the attention that is increasingly appropriated and privatized, despite our common claim to it" (Mariotti 2020, 488). She suggests that modern articulations of Zen meditation resonate with the thought of some political theorists of democracy, like Rancière, who emphasizes "momentary and reconfigurative fractures and fissures" that "throw some kind of grit in the gears of our conventional modes of perception, reorienting it and—in this dislocation and reconfiguration—also point toward alternatives" (477).

Such attempts to apply meditative practices to social and political reconfiguration are a significant development in the long history of Buddhist and Buddhist-derived meditative practices. They are happening, moreover, not just at a theoretical level but also on the ground.

Some examples:

A Barre Center for Buddhist Studies course:

What gets left out? Expanding Practice, Community, and Freedom. July 2020. Join Sebene Selassie & Brian Lesage in investigating some of the cultural frameworks (including patriarchy, colonialism, and norms of modernity) that we bring to our study and practice of Buddhism. Examine how these frameworks shape what is included and what gets left out.[3]

A meditation retreat at Spirit Rock, cosponsored by the East Bay Meditation Center:

White and Awakening Together
Crystal Johnson, PhD & Kitsy Schoen, MSW
8 Sundays, August 2–September 20, 10:00 a.m.–12:30 p.m. PT

This is a time in America when white people's awareness of the terrible impact of racial injustice has increased dramatically in the context of the pandemic and following the murders of George Floyd, Ahmaud Arbery and Breonna Taylor. How can we respond? What can we do? What is whiteness, and how does it fit in with our dharma practice? How can we use the energy of this time to explore and address the suffering of racial injustice and promote, nurture and maintain greater inclusiveness and racial equity in our communities?

Living in the U.S. (and elsewhere), we have been shaped by social, economic and other systems in which unearned privilege accrues to white people. To the extent that we are unaware of this system of white privilege and racial conditioning, we are not free to make skillful choices about how to live our values in the world. Rather, we unwittingly behave in ways that lead to suffering for ourselves, our community and the larger society. Further, we may not realize how our conditioning makes us resistant to joining with other white people to change the system and ourselves.

White and Awakening Together is designed as a guided, collaborative exploration of our racial conditioning as white people. We will apply dharma practices to explore the (un)realities of whiteness, stay present with difficult experiences and enhance our capacity to skillfully be in diverse community. Through this collaboration, we will expand our shared capacity to help each other learn and grow in ways that support liberation for us all.[4]

An online course from One Earth Sangha:

EcoSattva Training
An Online Course for Aspiring EcoSattvas

In the backdrop of a pandemic and state actors actively hostile to science, ecological breakdown looms. The potential for overwhelm, becoming captured by fear, rage, or helplessness, is real. While we take steps to demand racial justice, protect voting rights, or defend ecosystems, we can also invest in our inner resources. By integrating our activist dimensions with the contemplative, our efforts will be all the more robust and disentangled from reactivity. Turning towards what is profoundly difficult, supported by community, and transforming into wisdom is what this tradition is all about. Supported by a diverse and rich set of teachers, we invite you to gather with others online and explore our respective edges, meeting all that arises in us and discovering an authentic way forward.[5]

Such programmatic activities suggest an understanding of the autonomy that meditation can foster as expanding not only psychological conditions for personal liberation but also addressing the systemic conditions that make such autonomy possible. In such cases there is little pretense to neutrality or to an objective, value-free, nonjudgmental observation of interior facts. There is, instead, an explicit emphasis on particular ethical, social, and political values. Meditation in this case is used as an aid to deconstruct systems (both interior and societal) with values considered harmful and to actualize systems with better values. Here the affordances offered internally inevitably spill over into the external world, as meditators ask about what their society affords people with regard to their social and material conditions.

Social and Political Affordances

Affordances cannot be limited simply to the bare mechanics of organisms' relations with the physical environment. Any society brims with affordances that are available in different ways to different people. In any class structure, certain things are accessible to certain people and not to others. This is based on financial realities—one person literally can't afford things that another can—which often reflect structural advantages and disadvantages built into the system. Where I walk at night, where I drive, how I speak to different people, what products or foods I am drawn to or are available to me—all of these are structured by the "external" affordance landscape built in to a social structure. And they may well be quite different for a white, middle-aged, middle-class man (me) than they would be for a young, Black man. Cultural affordances in this sense are also socially available privileges—goods, services, activities are more accessible to one group rather than another.

Consideration of these issues has, for some practitioners, opened up possibilities of enlisting meditation not only in the relief of interior suffering but also of what Engaged Buddhists have called "systemic suffering." Thus meditators today interrogate the ways, for example, that the affordances one's society offers are unequally distributed or how environmental degradation curtails some peoples' life possibilities more than others. This model of meditative practice that examines not just "internal" but also systemic suffering is becoming more pervasive, as Dharma teachers increasingly attend to race, class, gender, economic inequality, and environmental issues as relevant to their contemplative analysis.

Such engagement with systemic suffering is not a given. Versions of the Inner Citadel model might approach these external affordance differentiations with the stance: they ultimately don't matter, they are only relative. What is important is my internal attitude, which is to maintain a certain detachment from them. If I am privileged—that is, if I experience a wide variety of cultural affordances, e.g., to food, material goods, social capital—then I *appreciate* the abundance available to me without getting too attached to it. If I am not as privileged, I can take comfort in the fact that these things do not matter so much or—in a more cosmologically inflected interpretation—do not reflect the ultimate, undifferentiated reality of things. What is causing my suffering is my *reactions* to these circumstances, thus my main task is to work with these reactions. The real truth of things is beyond the relative distinctions in the world, including (especially) personal and social identities—rich and poor, male and female, black and white. The one universal, underlying reality transcends all such distinctions, in this view.

In this attitude, the particular structures of secularism fuse with certain facets of Buddhism that accompany many contemporary applications of meditation. One element of secularism is that it purports to be a kind of neutral, value-free, transparent, universal mode of rational discourse. Indeed, it mirrors, and in some measure is based on, Kant's notion of disembedded rationality. And yet, again, to put it baldly, secularism isn't secular. That is, it is not a neutral space of free, rational thought and discourse unencumbered by the mythologies, superstitions, and irrational passions of "religion." Rather, it is itself a particular, culturally informed way of thinking, with a historical background, underlying assumptions, values, ideological components, and, indeed, mythologies, superstitions, and passions of its own. Secular iterations of Buddhist meditation often reproduce these features of secularism, including a certain blindness to the fact that it is itself a particular way of seeing, thinking, and feeling, rather than a neutral, value-free (nonjudgmental) mode of direct access to the truth. This is a stance that feels most natural to those already in a dominant social position within a secular society, a society in which their race, gender, or identity is not a barrier to that society's social affordances.

This is why meditators who attempt to apply their practice to social transformation and alleviating systemic suffering might put less emphasis on universalistic claims for meditation and more on the particulars of their ethical and social vision. They more unabashedly affirm the values and actions they wish to promote through meditation. Note, for example, how racial justice advocate and meditation teacher, Rhonda Magee, discussing how to apply mindfulness to racial issues, interprets being "nonjudgmental" in a way resonant with the distinction above between default morality and explicit ethics: "We will judge. But an important distinction mindfulness asks us to make is between automatic judgment and the more considered, deliberative evaluation that we might describe as *discernment*. This distinction is essential to the work of learning how to alleviate others' suffering, or of 'practicing justice'" (2019, 32).

As critics have suggested, versions of mindfulness that are bereft of any explicit ethical orientation might more easily assimilate themselves to mainstream values and support of the status quo because they are more likely to present the practice as transcending social particularities and "relative truths" in favor of universal ones. Yet, in this case, the "universal truths" they discover may simply be those that appear in a placid, accepting, nonjudgmental state and that promise not to disturb that tranquility. Meditation as an explicit excavation of default attitudes and orientations can be more unsettling and disruptive of tacit values. As the passage above suggests, work that applies a critical lens to the practitioner's interiority for specific purposes, such as overcoming unconscious racism, must engage conceptual thinking, apply particular values and judgments (or "discernments"), and make explicit one's implicit assumptions and attitudes. This approach might still be "secular" in the limited sense of "this-worldly," but it does not reproduce the implicit ideology of neutrality, the presumption of a thoroughly unbiased "view from nowhere" to which the secular gaze aspires. Instead, it acknowledges the specificity of suffering and employs meditation to help clarify how to alleviate it.

Conclusions on Meditation, Autonomy, and Ethics

The foundations of ethical agency are more complex than can be encapsulated by the axes of external versus internal or conformity and obedience versus personal freedom and autonomous choice. All of us inhabit complex, multiple, and intersecting social imaginaries that require selective affirmation, resistance, and adaptation. Meditative practices can be conducive to a sense of freedom and enhanced agency insofar as they bring to explicit consciousness what is normally tacit, whether these are motivations, affective states, dynamics of interpersonal relations, or frameworks through which we understand and move through the world, including social and political systems. Drawing these forth into the light of explicit consciousness opens up new affordances—new possibilities for interpretation, reflection, and action. Meditative practices can work both within and against available social imaginaries and their embedded ethical orientations, often navigating tensions between them. They may support dominant power structures or challenge them. They secure no guaranteed access to irrefutable truth, but rather, afford the possibility for clearer deliberation and navigation of the ethical dilemmas that face individuals in a social and political context.

I have addressed the Ethic of Autonomy as it relates to meditation, first, as a historical and cultural matter. Then, I have argued that the Situated Autonomy model is a more viable account of how meditation relates to agency than the Inner Citadel model. Yet there is something undeniably salient in the Inner Citadel approach that cannot be swept away casually, so let me, finally, put in a qualified good word for it. It is often said in contemporary meditation communities that "suffering is optional," a matter solely of internal orientation. You may not be able to control the fact that you became paralyzed, that you grew up poor, or that your husband left you. With the help of meditation, however, you *are* in control of your reactions to these situations. There is a point to this assertion, and indeed to the Inner Citadel side of the spectrum, which has been affirmed by Buddhist, Stoic, and other therapeutic philosophies and psychologies: people can cultivate flexibility in how to interpret and respond to unchosen or unalterable circumstances. Accepting what cannot be changed can indeed be liberating. Meditation works directly with these responses, creating what Buddhist literature calls "malleability of mind" (*citta-muduta*) by loosening up the interpretive potentials in any moment, helping meditators recognize that there is, perhaps, no final, locked-in meaning to any event. This pliancy might reveal the fecund hermeneutic potential of phenomena and help the practitioner avoid latching obsessively onto fixed interpretations. Thus meditation may provide ways of mitigating the sense of being thoroughly controlled by circumstances, thereby increasing one's agentive possibilities. Many activists who see meditation as a part of their activism cultivate this sense of an invulnerable interior space as a part of a necessary defense against the stresses that creating social and political change inevitably entail.

Nevertheless, uncompromising versions of the Inner Citadel model tend to disregard unchosen circumstances, social issues, material conditions— race, class, age, ethnicity, etc., as "external" or inessential factors in pursuit of internal peace. One's happiness or unhappiness is all a matter of what is happening inside one's head. For example: "Advocates of mindfulness would not accept in the first place the idea . . . that some actions, processes and outcomes in the world, including enhanced material welfare and the political strife it may entail, are superior to others. It is this idea, mindfulness maintains, which leads the fevered and benighted mind to clutch at them, supposing salvation to lie only in their attainment. For the serenely aware proponents of mindfulness, as for the ancient Greek Stoics, everything in the world is equal."[6] Relegating all meaning and significance to personal insights or choices ("choose happiness!") made within the mind, to the exclusion of all "external" circumstances, can devolve into a template that holds individuals so completely responsible for their own happiness and well-being that it appears fatalistic or indifferent to the undeniable importance of material, social, and structural realities, not to mention psychological factors or illness that may not be able to be reined in solely by meditation.

Working out the distinctions between "interior" and "exterior" and their implications has been a theme throughout our investigations. Much in the three ethical ideals we have looked at so far—appreciation, authenticity, and autonomy—tend toward individualism, with echoes of a bounded Cartesian self. In the next chapter, we examine how what I call the Ethic of Interdependence, a countervailing force, has emerged as part of an attempt to renegotiate this ever-ambiguous boundary, as well as the ethical demands of an interconnected world.

12

Individualism and Fragmentation in the Mirrors of Secularism

The Ethic of Interdependence

Dispatches from the Worlds of Meditation: 12

All the myriad phenomena before his eyes—the old and the young, the honorable and the base, halls and pavilions, verandahs and corridors, plants and trees, mountains and rivers—he regards as his own original, true, and pure aspect. It is just like looking into a bright mirror and seeing his own face in it. If he continues for a long time to observe everything everywhere with this radiant insight, all appearances of themselves become the jeweled mirror of his own house, and he becomes the jeweled mirror of their houses as well.

—Hakuin Ekaku, 1686–1769

Hand Mirrors and Infinity Mirrors

Consider two works of art featuring mirrors. The first, by Thomas Worlidge (1700–1766), a British painter and etcher, is titled "A Portrait of a Young Man, William Taylor, Looking in a Mirror" (Figure 12.1). The etching is precisely what its title promises: a man looking into a small hand mirror, which reflects his puffy visage and buoyantly coiffed hair. It makes an apt emblem of the European Enlightenment, whose philosophers promised to develop the methods that would hold man and nature up to the mirror of empirical investigation and rational analysis, rendering clear and distinct representations of them. Nothing else appears in the work but the young man, his mirror, and his reflection.

The contemporary Japanese artist Yayoi Kusama offers a very different mirror-themed work, a series called Infinity Mirror Rooms (Figure 12.2). In one, a viewer stands in a room whose walls are mirrors reflecting uncountable numbers of lights receding in all directions. Although a small room, it seems

Rethinking Meditation. David L. McMahan, Oxford University Press. © Oxford University Press 2023.
DOI: 10.1093/oso/9780197661741.003.0012

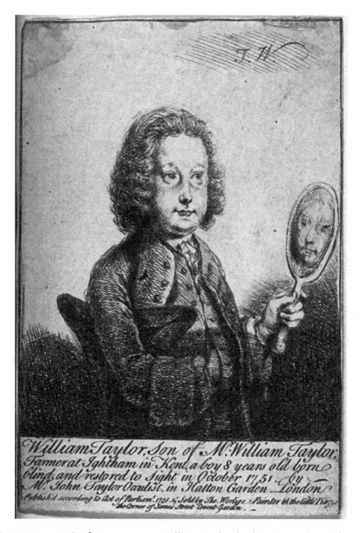

FIGURE 12.1 A portrait of a young man, William Taylor, looking in a mirror. Thomas Worlidge, 1751.

enormous, indeed infinite, and includes multiple images of the viewer herself. People around the world wait in line for hours to stand in these rooms and experience themselves enveloped in countless lights and objects multiplied throughout unlimited space.

If Worlidge's image was compelling in the eighteenth century for illustrating the Enlightenment ideal of the mirror of nature and the promise of clear and accurate representation of the autonomous, independent individual, Kusama's image is more resonant with our age and its fragmentation, its conscious-ness of the vastness of the cosmos, and its hope for some significance—some

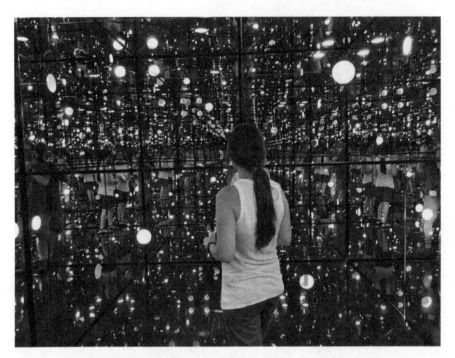

FIGURE 12.2 Yayoi Kusama, *Infinity Mirrored Room—Illusion Inside the Heart*, 2020, New York Botanical Garden. Photo by David McMahan.

reflection of ourselves—in that vastness. We might consider the two images suggestive of two archetypal ways of considering—or perhaps experiencing— oneself in the world. One, a coherent sense of selfhood, distinct from the world and clear to itself, still echoes in our time in calls for authenticity, self-realization, individualism, identity, thinking for oneself. The other represents a contemporary sense of multiple, displaced, disembedded, vertiginous subjectivity, more difficult to pin down, more disorienting and perhaps frightening, but also potentially expansive and ecstatic.

These images illustrate competing versions of secular subjectivity. Although the Infinity Mirror version is more recent, the hand mirror version is by no means a relic of the past. We might instead see the contemporary era as marked by a tension between the two. In this chapter, I want to consider how particular elements of the *zeitgeist* of secularity have drawn forth and transformed certain specific elements of Buddhism—especially the doctrine of nonself (*anātman*), dependent origination or interdependence (*pratītya-samutpāda*), and certain meditative practices. These elements of Buddhism, I suggest, have been transformed in ways that both embrace and attempt to ameliorate certain ills of contemporary secularity as a lived experience. More specifically, they attempt to negotiate the tension between the two modes of modern secular subjectivity suggested by our two mirror-themed works of art: the sense of selfhood as singular, independent, and autonomous and the sense of fragmentation of the self into multiple identities.

Modernity and the Fragmentation of the Self

Here is a brief story about the experience of selfhood in the modern West, how it developed and changed, and how it prepared the ground for particular versions of Buddhism to emerge. It is a ridiculously abbreviated and too-neat story, and we could fill a book with caveats and attempts to nuance it, but we can't, so here it is. The Age of Enlightenment promised a kind of narrative clarity about the self. Descartes claimed to isolate the soul definitively—"I am nothing but a thinking thing." At its best, the soul or self, had "clear and distinct" ideas. The discovery (or creation) of this self was part of a larger "subjective turn" in the West, through which attention turned inward as never before in European history (Taylor 1989). The subjective turn entailed attempts to systematically account for the faculties of mind and body, nail them down, establish once and for all just what the soul of man (yes, man) was and its place in the universe. The Enlightenment thinkers proposed that rationality was the essence of the self, and that through stepping away from the emotions and relying solely on reason, one could make moral choices and live a good life. Romanticism countered this notion by insisting on the centrality of emotion, of passion, of deep interiority, of getting in touch with nature and the divine through interior exploration. Although they seem opposed, these two versions of selfhood were complementary and shared the notion of the autonomous individual whose judgment could, and should, transcend social convention and be the sole author of itself. We can characterize these visions of selfhood as "secular" not because they necessarily rejected God or divinity altogether but because they shifted emphasis from dependence on God to self-determination and individual autonomy.

　　Charles Taylor argues that a distinctive characteristic of this newly constituted modern self is that it is "buffered" rather than porous. That is, the modern West inaugurated a firmer boundary between the self and objects than had existed in the premodern, enchanted world. In the enchanted world, he claims, this boundary was porous, and people were more vulnerable to the influences of external things—gods, spirits, and demons—directly. Objects were charged with inherent meaning: black bile was not just a physical cause of melancholy as a mental state—it *was* melancholy. Sand from a sacred place could have beneficent, healing effects—the sand *itself*, not just the salutary effects on the mind of believing in healing sand. This is not just a matter of beliefs but of a deep-rooted way of experiencing and interpreting oneself and the world. Think also of the significance of dreams or hearing voices in a lot of ancient literature: one heard God's voice; or maybe it's that of a demon. Today, although many people still gather sand from sacred sites, see ghosts, and hear voices, most of us experience such things within the framework of a bounded self—the mind, the inside—more distinct from the external world. If I see a ghost, I wonder if it might be an eruption of my unconscious, a repressed memory, a hallucination, or the result of a chemical imbalance. I might explain any beneficent effect of sacred sand in terms of the effect it has on my mood; or perhaps it's a kind of placebo effect. In the buffered self, the mind is the locus of all meaning, and the external world in itself is the blank slate for the projections of meanings. This framework also makes for the possibility of distancing oneself from the manifestations of the mind and treating them as objects—observing, controlling, and disciplining them (Taylor 2007, 2008). The point is that the autonomous individual of the Enlightenment philosophers was a theoretical expression of something that was also taking shape on a more phenomenological level among many people in the West. If Descartes's "thinking thing" was a dry philosophical abstraction, it was (if Taylor is right) also refracted in the ordinary experience of "buffered selves" who, encouraged by educational and institutional structures, began more and more to conceive of and experience themselves as enclosed, self-contained beings with private minds separate from the world.

I have some reservations about drawing a firm line between a premodern "enchanted world" and the modern "disenchanted world,"[1] but there does seem to be something, as I mentioned in chapter 1, to the idea that modern, western people experience themselves as having a firmer boundary between inside and outside than those in other cultures and historical periods. If it is true that a novel sense of self-enclosed subjectivity gradually emerged in the modern period, we might characterize late modernity—the latter half of the twentieth to the present—as a period when this sense of the autonomous, buffered self begins to fray at the edges. Countless examples from philosophy, art, literature, sociology, psychology, and religious studies might offer insights into this. I only offer a few gleanings.

Social theorist Anthony Giddens marks "late" or "high" modernity as a period of increased disembeddedness from traditional social orders in which people's roles are more rigidly defined. Rather than a being embedded in a family, community, social order, and cosmos that gives a de facto meaning to their lives, people in the conditions of late modernity are increasingly thrown back on themselves to continuously figure out and construct who they are. The self, in other words, becomes a "reflexive project":

> Transitions in individuals' lives have always demanded psychic reorganisation, something which was often ritualised in traditional cultures in the shape of *rites de passage*. But in such cultures, where things stayed more or less the same from generation to generation on the level of the collectivity, the changed identity was clearly staked out—as when an individual moved from adolescence into adulthood. In the settings of modernity, by contrast, the altered self has to be explored and constructed as part of a reflexive process of connecting personal and social change. (1991, 32–3)

Such conditions, Giddens argues, create increased uncertainty and doubt, as well as a sense of the fragility of one's narrative of the self. "A self-identity has to be created and more or less continually reordered against the backdrop of shifting experiences of day-to-day life and the fragmenting tendencies of modern institutions" (186). In premodern times, Giddens argues, people's identities were, to a great extent, determined by gender, family, clan, lineage, and so on. Today some of these factors are still important; however, people increasingly must actively construct identities through "lifestyles," consumer choices, and interaction with many abstract systems, such as the educational system, the healthcare system, and the ubiquitous economic system of global capitalism. One must continually construct and revise one's identity in multiple contexts, repeatedly adapting and creating a "narrative of self"—a coherent life story that appears to maintain itself throughout time. According to Giddens, the splintering of the self, and the energy-consuming struggle to maintain a sense of narrative coherence, can lead to a disorienting sense of fragmentation, uncertainty, doubt, and the looming threat of personal meaninglessness.

Zygmunt Bauman extends some of Giddens's insights on the malleability of the self in the contemporary era. He characterizes the contemporary period as one of "liquid life" in which conditions change at such a rapid rate that predicting the future on the basis of the past becomes increasingly difficult and, therefore, anxiety-producing. It is a period in which people, rather than having an identity given to them at birth based on being embedded in family, community, and nation, must create their identities in an ad hoc fashion. Baumann highlights the differential effects this situation has on people in different socioeconomic strata:

At the top [of the social hierarchy], the problem is to choose the best pattern from the many currently on offer, to assemble the separately sold parts of the kit, and to fasten them together neither too lightly (lest the unsightly, outdated and aged bits that are meant to be hidden underneath show through at the seams) nor too tightly (lest the patchwork resists being dismantled at short notice when the time for dismantling comes—as it surely will). At the bottom, the problem is to cling fast to the sole identity available and to hold its bits and parts together while fighting back the erosive forces and disruptive pressures, repairing the constantly crumbling walls and digging the trenches deeper. (2005, 6)

Identity must be constantly constructed, reconstructed, and maintained in large part through consumption of items—cars, phones, décor, clothing—of limited life and temporary value in conferring cultural capital. The self itself then comes to feel tenuous, fleeting, unstable, and thus continually in need of scrutiny and reform, while the external world is reduced to having primarily instrumental value. Individuality, rather than a given of our nature, as assumed by both the Enlightenment and Romantic thinkers, is an endless task to be achieved through lifelong struggle amid dizzyingly rapid change. For Baumann, achieving individuality, therefore, is an "*aporia*"—an irresolvable contradiction— in a society that demands uniqueness and yet has undercut the social bonds of community that would confer any sense of stable identity. Thus, Baumann claims, "the struggle for *uniqueness* has now become the main engine of *mass* production and *mass* consumption" (Baumann 2005, 24). Identity is perpetually hybrid, unstable, unfixed, yet always promised. And yet the construction of identity through career and consumer choice remains a privilege for those who can afford it, while those in less privileged sectors of society remain stuck in assigned, imposed, "over-determined" identity (26). No one escapes "liquid modernity," however: the affluent global, "deterritorialized" citizen learns to ride the waves of rapid change while the underprivileged struggle with the risk of constantly being left behind, bereft of economic and cultural capital.

Psychologist Kenneth Gergen adds to this picture the ways that "technologies of social saturation"—primarily media technologies—have contributed to the sense of self-fragmentation:

Emerging technologies saturate us with the voices of humankind—both harmonious and alien. As we absorb their varied rhymes and reasons, they become a part of us and we of them. Social saturation furnishes us with a multiplicity of incoherent and unrelated languages of the self. For everything we "know to be true" about ourselves, other voices within respond with doubt and even derision. This fragmentation of self-conceptions corresponds to a multiplicity of incoherent and disconnected relationships. These relationships pull us in myriad directions, inviting us to play such a variety of roles that the very concept of an "authentic self" with knowable characteristics recedes from view. The fully saturated self becomes no self at all. (2000, 7)

As we are bombarded with ever-multiplying social contexts, the languages of the self inherited from modernism and romanticism—the knowable, rational, autonomous individual and the passionate soul with a deep interior—begin to recede. If, in the past, a sense of relatively stable selfhood was created by embeddedness in tightknit communities with relatively stable roles, the "saturated self" confronts countless others—physical, fictional, virtual—and is called on to respond to each, creating a sense of subjectivity characterized by "a plurality of voices all vying for the right to reality" (Gergen 2000, 7). The world of rapid travel and instant communication has created, Gergen argues, a situation in which "we are bombarded with ever increasing intensity with the images and actions of others; our range of social participation is increasing exponentially." In this world, "we no longer experience a secure sense of self," and "doubt is increasingly placed on the very assumption of a bounded identity with palpable attributes" (15–16).

Social saturation brings with it a general loss in our assumption of true and knowable selves. As we absorb multiple voices, we find that each "truth" is relativized by our simultaneous consciousness of compelling alternatives. We come to be aware that each truth about ourselves is a construction of the moment, true only for a given time and within certain relationships. (16)

Gergen dubs the "infusion of partial identities through social saturation" the "populated self," a cacophony of images and voices representing disparate possibilities of selfhood that are constantly displaced by others. This condition is not merely a matter of self-concepts but also of activities and investments of time and energy. One effect is what he calls "multiphrenia . . . the splitting of the individual into a multiplicity of self-investments" (73–4). The expansion of relationships leads to the "vertigo of the valued," in which each context of interaction entails new things to value, desire, and choose, until life becomes a vertiginous swirl of beckonings and demands.

Now we shouldn't be so naïve as to think that this collage of late-modern subjectivities amounts to something all-encompassing or universal. Although there is little doubt that, while the symptoms they describe have gone global, they may be refracted quite differently in different cultural, class, or gender contexts, and may even be relatively absent in some. There is also reason for some skepticism about Taylor's distinction between "porous" and "buffered" selves. People today still hear the voice of God and experience various enchantments and mysteries that many educated people have relegated to the "premodern" past but are still quite alive today (Luhrmann 2020). No doubt, further nuancing is needed, but for now let's hazard the generalizations that, first, the modern world brought forth not just new ideas of individualism but also a felt sense of experiencing the world in a more bounded way, as an individual mind separate from an objective world; and second, that the conditions of late modernity have encouraged a sense of subjective fragmentation that disrupts the sense of the modern autonomous individual, as well as more "premodern" embeddedness in communities. Most pertinent to Buddhism in the West, these phenomena were likely familiar to those who have been responsible for bringing Buddhism into North America and Europe as a live option throughout the late twentieth century. Whether they have been Japanese immigrant priests, Tibetan refugee lamas, or educated and spiritually curious European Americans, those who have shaped modern Buddhism have either experienced or been keen observers of this new mode of secular consciousness.

So the picture that coalesces from these authors about contemporary modes of subjectivity in the West is that the "modern self," with its valorization of self-reliance, individual autonomy, and freedom from the external coercion is splintering. In hindsight, it was always deeply flawed as a theory, but as an ideologically driven phenomenological sense of self, it attained a kind of provisional actuality as a coherent constellation of habits, dispositions, and sensibilities. Therefore, its splintering in the face of the above factors forms a part of the topography of late-modern anxiety, stress, and malaise. There is, then, a tension at work in late-modern secular subjectivities, especially in the West: the modern construction of the self-sufficient, self-responsible, free agent separate from the objective world, isolated and buffered—a lingering centripetal force of Enlightenment individualism—exists in tension with a centrifugal sense of internal fragmentation, media saturation, rootlessness, and disembeddedness. The late-modern secular subject, with the Enlightenment inheritance still part of the background understanding of individualistic personhood, retains this self-understanding as an ideal, even when it is threatened daily by the forces of fragmentation. The man looking at his singular reflection in the hand mirror begins to see his image distort, double, triple, then explode into an infinity of images, some of himself, some of others, all scattering into a dizzying array of lights expanding to infinity.

How is it, then, that various strands of Buddhist thought and practice weave their way into this picture and create a further chapter in the story? How are certain elements of Buddhism and its meditative practices envisioned as either accommodating this sense of subjectivity or offering ameliorative, transformative possibilities for its ills?

Fragmented Selves and Nonself

The secularization of Buddhism is a process more complex than "Buddhism" being imported into "Western culture" or "modern culture" or any other singular thing. Different selected threads of Buddhisms around the world have been reconfigured and woven into the fabric of a globalized secular modernity (which is itself really an extended family of modernities and secularities, not all of which are "western"), while other threads have been ignored. How could it be otherwise? So rather than list the various solutions and possibilities that Buddhism may offer to the tension between individualism and fragmentation I've outlined above, I confine myself to considering some secular interpretations of particular Buddhist ideas and practices: the ideas of nonself and interdependence, and the practice of contemporary meditation. I am not suggesting that these ideas and practices stand on their own as true and efficacious per se, and therefore provide solutions to the conditions I've identified. Rather, I am looking historically at how these social conditions (along with others) have created a space for certain Buddhist ideas and practices and have drawn them forth out of their home contexts and into new habitations of late-modern secularity.

The most obvious place to begin is with the Buddhist insistence on the absence of an independent, enduring, and unchanging self (*ātman*). Given the received notions of modern western selfhood rooted in the Enlightenment and Romanticism, the prospects for the doctrine of nonself (*anātman*) in the West would seem dim. But nonself functions in particular ways when drawn into the orbit of late-modern secular subjectivity and its chaotic liquidity, media saturation, instability, disembeddedness, and fragmentation—not to mention the nostalgia for the stable, self-responsible agent of the Enlightenment.

If Giddens and Bauman are right that many people in late modernity are disembedded from the social forces that provided a ready-made identity and that, instead, we must now constantly ask "who am I?"—that identity is not given and so requires a continuing task of constructing a stable, narrative self—then certain interpretations of *anātman* become, for some, a compelling way of navigating this reality. If we have never had a coherent, stable, permanent self to begin with, then attempting to construct one is not only unnecessary but futile. Following this logic, it is better to recognize the fluid, malleable nature of consciousness, be aware of how various "selves" rise and fall depending on diverse causes and conditions, and learn to skillfully guide the process. This approach might serve to mitigate the anxiety of trying to anchor a stable sense of selfhood amid the whirlwind of ever-changing conditions of the late-modern period. If the bad news for the modern autonomous self is that it was a fiction to begin with—something that philosophy, psychology, neuroscience, and social science increasingly agree on—the good news is that a rich, meaningful, and ethical life is available in its absence. If the fragmenting forces of late modernity have shattered the illusion of a fixed self, *anātman* provides a way of rethinking subjectivity in its absence.

The doctrine of *anātman* claims that, in the face of the constant flux of plural selves "vying for the right to reality," as Gergen puts it, that none actually has such a right. In a time of the multiplication of self-images and frantic attempts to ground one of them in reality, refiguring subjectivity as nonself accepts that such grounding will never happen and, moreover, that abandoning the attempt is part of the solution to the problem. And yet there is the possibility of agency and intention outside the confines of the isolated, autonomous self. *Anātman* introduces a way to imagine navigating the tensions between, on the one hand, the Cartesian notion of the bounded, autonomous self and, on the other hand, the lived experience of fragmentation, saturation, and permeability of the self. The autonomous self, it suggests, is a fiction. We are a combination of various processes coming together under the influence of past actions that color, constitute, and characterize the present. Yet we have agency, in each moment, for further directing this complex process, our own stream of consciousness, in more wise and compassionate directions. In this view, we are neither wholly determined by the past nor fully free from it.

Two Poles of Mindfulness

Reimagining subjectivity in this way is intimately intertwined with secular adaptations of Buddhist meditative practices. If the splintering of subjectivity into multiple selves, commitments, and projects constitutes a uniquely modern anxiety, what new uses and transformations of mindfulness emerge in the space created by these conditions? First, we can see mindfulness as the detached observation of these "selves" and their activities, which may dereify them, decrease anxiety, and lessen the feeling of being trapped by them or overwhelmed by their mercurial flux, allowing room for critical reflection on the process. Rather than fleeing the modern burden of hyperreflexivity that Giddens outlines, meditative practices plunge the practitioner into the process in order to observe and reconfigure it. Mindfulness promises to harness the fragmented sense of self, cull it into a manageable, intention-directed stream of consciousness, and conjure a sense of steadiness—even resoluteness—out of the infinitely plural phenomenological continuum.

Given this interpretation, though, meditative practices might gravitate toward either of two poles. They might be used to shore up the "buffered self" and reassert the ebbing sense of autonomous selfhood. Popular culture in the United States and Europe (and increasingly around the world) tells us that we, indeed, have a self that we need to discover, and to do this we need to look within. When we discover who we are, we must be true to that self, casting off socially conditioned influences to emerge as a truly free, autonomous, and self-contained being. As we have seen, some approaches to mindfulness implicitly take up this approach, using contemplative methods originally designed to undermine the perception of a fixed, permanent self, to reinforce the individualism so deeply rooted in western culture. They attempt to strike back against fragmentation by using meditation to re-affirm the integrated, singular individual—the man in the mirror. In this sense, meditation, mindfulness, self-monitoring, and self-observation have the potential to exacerbate the sense of individual isolation, separation from the world, and even narcissism. These interpretations of mindfulness tend to be either purely introspective or instrumental, offering either private psychological comfort or increasing effectiveness at doing whatever one happened to be doing anyway. If mindfulness is a tool to enhance the efficiency of the autonomous self, then it can, in the current context, simply reinforce a sense of isolated individuality, to which instrumentalized, decontextualized, commercialized, and corporatized applications of mindfulness become an appendage.

The other pole of interpretation retains something more substantive from the Buddhist tradition and uses contemplative methods to deconstruct the singular identity, to recognize the radical impermanence and multiplicity of conscious experience, and to open up the buffered self—not to the spirits and demons of old, but to a renewed sense of connection and interwovenness with the world. This approach might mitigate the forces of fragmentation not by retreating to a doubly bounded and isolated subjectivity but by admitting the open, fluid, multiple nature of human consciousness and its intimate relatedness to other individuals, to community, to the physical objects in our lives, and to the natural and built worlds we inhabit.

There is, therefore, a tension between two poles of interpretation of modern, secular mindfulness practices: at one pole is mindfulness as a private matter, a matter of personal experience and psychological health or instrumental efficiency; on the other is mindfulness as an awakening to a more urgent sense of connectedness with others, which in turn may foster particular ethical sensibilities. These approaches are all interfused with secularity insofar as they take for granted the value of *this* world instead of striving for another. They mostly accept the modern naturalistic worldview, which shifts attention away from otherworldly aims—eternal bliss in nirvana, rebirth in the Pure Land—in favor of this-worldly projects. One pole is constituted by a combination of various elements of Buddhism—self-discipline and karmic responsibility, for example—with the of picture of the autonomous self derived from secular modernism and neoliberalism, with its emphasis on personal choice, self-responsibility, independence, and self-determination. The other combines other elements of Buddhism—compassion for all sentient beings, interdependence or (in some cases) oneness of self and world—with a greater emphasis on a political, social, and ecological ethic emphasizing systemic suffering and care for the world and other beings. Secularity, with its shift to this-worldly concerns, provides the scaffolding for both poles of this continuum, and the many possibilities in between.

Secularity and Interdependence

These reimaginings of subjectivity through the idea of nonself, as well as the contemporary interpretations of mindfulness I've mentioned, negotiate the issue of the interior and exterior, the individual and the social, that we have been tracing throughout this book; and they are intimately related to modern articulations of the classical Buddhist doctrine of interdependence. The resurgence and rethinking of the ancient doctrine of dependent arising (*pratītya-samutpāda*) is perhaps inevitable in today's world, in which interconnectivity is the undeniable blessing and curse of the age. Contemporary interconnectedness allows the grandmother in Taiwan to talk in real time to her grandson in Evansville, Illinois, and the carpet-buyer in Los Angeles to put money in the pocket of the sweatshop owner in Pakistan. It allows feminism, white nationalism, lithium batteries, and CO_2 to pervade the globe with ease and speed unimaginable even a generation ago. Contemporary notions of interdependence extend to the cosmic realm, as humanity gets used to the recently discovered fact of the near unimaginable vastness of the universe. Thus, it is no wonder that people wait in line for hours to stand in Kusama's Infinity Mirror Rooms in order to feel the expansive sense of themselves and their world in countless reflected images mingling and trailing off into endlessness. Art reviewers have noticed the relevance of the Infinity Mirror rooms to Buddhism. In his review of one installation, Michael Venables suggests that it invokes the Buddhist doctrine of emptiness and Thich Nhat Hanh's "interbeing," a popular modern articulation of the doctrine of dependent arising:

> Thinking about Kusama's art, I find the Buddhist concept of "emptiness" to be useful. First, we are all uncertain expressions of a world that is passing. It begins with your own realization of the great cloud of dots, of which you are a part: your own "emptiness of essence." . . . Might this be something akin to Thich Nhat Hanh's "interbeing"? An affirmation of the inter-connectedness of the essence of all things? . . . It's the experience of infinity, in an instant of time. A sense of place in what seems like the chaos of our modern world. It's a feeling of hope, of connecting the Kusama dots that can bind us all together.[2]

Venables' drawing together Kusama's Infinity Mirror rooms with Nhat Hanh's formulation of interbeing gestures toward a particular modern understanding of interdependence as a way of enchanting the world. His poetic descriptions of the cloud in the paper (the cloud produces rain, which waters the tree, which provides material for the paper) or the mutual dependence of roses and garbage (the rose depends on decomposing material to nourish it, then it dies and becomes compost for other plants) provide mundane examples of how things exist in a vast process of mutually interdependent events. We too, are a part of this process of the cosmos producing innumerable forms, transforming into each other in a boundless web of interconnected life. In this view, "I" am not this limited form but rather the entire process; the whole ocean and not merely this one temporary wave (Nhat Hanh 1988, 1991). Such images take the mundane stuff of life and weave them together in ways that strive at once to gently obliterate the fixed, independent self of the Enlightenment and ease the frenetic fragmentation of the saturated self through mindfulness. Or perhaps ease *into* that fragmentation and reinterpret it as communion with all things. Nhat Hanh's interbeing takes the raw ingredients of secular cosmology and infuses them with wonder by imagining the re-opening of the isolated self into the cosmos, a reintegration into the alienated world, an expansion of the I into all things. But he offers nothing to transgress the basic foundations of the discourse of naturalistic secularity—no rebirth in the traditional sense, no heavens or hells, no miracles except mindfully walking on the earth. His unbufferring of secular subjectivity invites in no demons or gods or voices from other worlds. Just clouds, paper, roses, garbage, stars, planets, and each other.

Modern interpretations of interdependence like this take the splintered and decentered and reconfigure it as expansive and grand. They negotiate ways in which the fraying of the self-contained individual, with its scattering across so many spheres of activity, obligation, and meaning, can be called to order as a beautiful, expansive interwovenness with the cosmos. Rather than experiencing the world as a network of hostile forces aligned against an individual self, on the one hand, or as an overwhelming array of ever-splintering selves, on the other, one is invited to imagine all things as contiguous with oneself. Your current form is just one of many that you will take. The *you* that you think is you is not you—the real you is everything. Nhat Hanh's cosmos is not a cold, lifeless, indifferent world receding into nothingness but a living process tossing up form after form in a playful, creative, and infinite unfolding. Such a view offers an enchanted cosmology that affirms the truths of scientific naturalism, with its webs of life and complex systems, giving them a glow of mystery and wholeness.

Contemporary Buddhists may think that this vision of interdependence has been in place in Buddhist thought all along. It hasn't. In early Buddhism, the interdependent world of *saṃsāra* was not a wondrous web of life but a binding chain, a "mass of suffering" from which one must escape. Mahāyāna ideas emerged, however, that would provide resources for rethinking the value of the phenomenal world. If nirvana and *saṃsāra* are not different, as Nāgārjuna asserted, awakening could be interpreted as a matter of seeing the world aright rather than escaping it altogether. And the bodhisattva vow—to postpone exiting the world until all sentient beings have become awakened— is, in effect, a commitment to remain in *saṃsāra* indefinitely. In Tantric traditions and in East Asia, *saṃsāra* also got rehabilitated in some measure. As the doctrine of buddha-nature expanded to nature itself, Chinese Buddhist thinkers began to think of it as infusing the natural world, wrapping a pre-existing reverence for mountains and rivers into Buddhist intuitions. When Buddhism came West, this reverence was woven into the Transcendentalist thought of Emerson and Thoreau, with their valorization of nature and pan-theistic inclinations. This, in turn, paved the way for thinking of the interdependent world in a time of globalization and climate change as a wondrous and fragile web of connection for which we all have ethical responsibility.[3]

Nevertheless, if modern articulations of interdependence like Nhat Hanh's are enchantments of secular interdependence, they are also secularizations of earlier Buddhist portrayals. Kusama's, in fact, are not the first infinity mirrors to emerge from Asia. The second-century Indian Buddhist text the

Gaṇḍavyūha Sūtra, part of the vast *Avataṃsaka Sūtra*, is an orgy of visionary imagery seemingly designed to disrupt the ordinary sense of self, space, and time through the infinite multiplication of images. In its climax, the main character, a pilgrim named Sudhana, encounters a great enlightened being, Samantabhadra. Rather than having a conversation, Sudhana gazes at him intently and sees that there are universes "as infinite as the sands of the Ganges" in each of the pores of his skin. And in each universe, Sudhana sees an image of himself (Cleary 1989, 386–7). Later, in China, the sixth-to seventh-century Huayan Buddhist philosopher, Fazang, attempted to boil down the narrative to a single image: reality is like a candle in a room with opposite-facing mirrors. Everything reflects and interpenetrates everything else, while still remaining distinct. Every individual contains the whole, and the whole is dependent on each individual. Another image used in Huayan Buddhism has become popular in recent ecological discussions: Indra's net—a net expanding out infinitely with a multifaceted reflecting jewel at each juncture. Each jewel in the net contains the mirror-image of all of the other jewels, while that single jewel is likewise reflected in all the others.

How is it that such images are drawn into the sensibilities of secular subjectivity and transformed by its hopes, fears, and anxieties? Like contemporary mindfulness, the Infinity Mirror model of self and world has variant possible interpretations. First is an aestheticized version of interdependence, focusing on wonder and comfort, blunting the edges of gritty physicality and shedding a soft-focus light on the harsh realities of death, illness, aging, and vulnerability to the capriciousness of the world. In this sense it may be comforting but potentially anaesthetizing of the reality that Buddhism itself has insisted we should look at squarely—remember the grizzly descriptions of the interiors of bodies and of corpses in the cremation ground.

Other possible interpretations exist, however. If the valorizing of wonder pushes human agency in the direction of passivity (things are beyond my personal control; death and suffering aren't so bad; or, perhaps, everything works together for a grand, cosmic good, so accept and surrender to it), other interpretations insist on ethical, social, and political implications. They urge action. It is no wonder that Indra's Net has become a recurring image in ecological and social thought, where it is a potent symbol for the densely interconnected biosphere or the fraying social fabric, both under threat. Shake one part of the net and the reverberations are projected throughout its entirety, like coal smoke from China reaching Alaska or ethnic nationalism in the United States coalescing with similar movements throughout Europe, spreading like wildfire across the internet.

Here the vision of intertwinement of self and world tends not (or at least not only) toward passive wonderment but also toward a heightened sense of ethical, social, and political responsibility. Infinite interconnectedness as an ethical imperative entails a recognition that all actions reverberate into the wider world. It opens up attention to the systemic suffering perpetrated by the webs of interactions inherent in the globalized economic and political spheres. It encourages re-envisionings of right livelihood to include, for example, the consumer choices of the wealthy and their effects on the lives of the poor and disenfranchised. Some contemporary Buddhist authors encourage a sense of empathy that fosters imagining oneself as the other, as all others—as everything—and taking responsibility for the world as one would a part of one's own body, a body extending infinitely outward (for example, Loy 2019, Kaza 2019, Macy 1991).

If I am right that there are tensions—creative and conflictual—between these different approaches to nonself, meditation, and interdependence, then underlying these tensions is perhaps the fundamental tension between versions of Buddhism as mainly a private matter—of personal experience, individual enlightenment, or psychological health—and Buddhism as more active and engaged in the monumental social, political, and ecological problems of the present age. This is by no means a stark, binary choice, and there is a spectrum of possibilities in between. Someone might simply use mindfulness for reducing stress, for example, but also be an avid political activist. But all of these approaches I've mentioned are interfused with secularity insofar as they take for granted the value of *this* world instead of striving for another.

Fractal Order and Fragmented Chaos

In his influential book, *Philosophy and the Mirror of Nature*, Richard Rorty describes the aspiration of modern philosophy and science to be a "mirror of nature," a "final language" that directly reflects and gives a definitive account of things as they are (1979). That battered ideal of the mirror of nature still survives today, mainly in the sciences, but in many ways it has given way to a funhouse mirror, where truth is harder to nail down, and competing versions of every conceivable thing multiply endlessly in ever-proliferating internet worlds. If there was ever a time when Thomas Worlidge's young man could gaze into his hand mirror and rest content in the singular vision of an uncomplicated individual self, that time has passed. Today we have multiple identities—personal, professional, legal, political, virtual. They are reflected back at us, in chaotic rapid-fire, in pixilated screens. Meanwhile, recent cosmology depicts humans as brief, accidental, and fragile wisps of living matter in an infinitely vast, impersonal universe. The dominant "strategy" of many Buddhists and Buddhist sympathizers in allowing Buddhism to speak to this situation has been to infuse selected Buddhist ideas, practices, and images into secular discourse, with the hope that they will whisper a sense of wonder within confusion, invoke fractal order out of fragmented chaos, and assert responsibility in the face of powerlessness. It remains to be seen whether these bits of Buddhism and its meditative traditions will be subsumed and tamed by secularism's more rapacious elements—commodification, commercialization, and trivialization—or have a significant transformative effect on the ethos of secularity itself.

Postscript: The Iron Age and the Anthropocene

The first dispatches from the worlds of meditation are lost to our gaze, well beyond our temporal horizons, before the teachings of the Buddha. It is unfashionable today to speculate on origins, yet it is tantalizing to imagine the first moments when people began to turn the mind's eye back on itself, to attend closely to sensations, flickerings of thought and desire, impressions, memories, the stream of words and sentences. And more, to attribute some significance to this procession, to consider that, perhaps, it held some secret, some mystery to be unlocked, some imperative to be followed; that it held even the possibility of transcendent freedom, of conquering death, of knowing where things come from and where they go, of knowing what one truly is. The Vedas suggest that the people who began such experiments were attempting to transpose the sacrifices to the gods to the internal realm, to kindle an internal fire through breath and imagination, sending the internalized oblations and prayers to the deities. This must have taken some effort to arrange thoughts, desires, and imagery, and for some, this introspective observation and ordering must have begun to take on a life of its own. From the gods' perspective, the turn toward attending to consciousness itself might have seemed a dangerous distraction, a move toward self-absorption rather than proper attentiveness to them. And the meditative path, in fact, did lead many away from the gods; its culmination was said to be "beyond the gods." So perhaps it is not so hard to see why some fragments of this path now renew themselves in a secular age.

It may be hard to think of ourselves today as the benefactors of these Iron Age experimenters. Today most people meditate not to get to some eternity beyond the gods but to create meaning and enchantment this side of them. But whatever modernity is, it is never a complete break with what has preceded it; perhaps it is the more frenetic reappropriation of the past, of its multiple threads winding down circuitously to weave their way into our present moments, beckoning us—challenging us—to make some sense of them. It is difficult to imagine that the college student sitting on folded pillows on his

Rethinking Meditation. David L. McMahan, Oxford University Press. © Oxford University Press 2023.
DOI: 10.1093/oso/9780197661741.003.0013

bed baffled by his own mind, or the woman sitting in a chair in the corporate boardroom letting go for a moment of her hectic schedule, or the activist sitting with legs crossed, blocking traffic at a busy intersection, as the inheritors of the intentional actions—literally, the *karma*—of the ancient ascetics who invented meditation. But indeed, these practices, transformed, reinvented, and rethought over and over again, have snaked their way through many cultural worlds down to ours. They have been called upon to help people escape to a world within, to help them kill others in war, to help them manage their scholarly productivity, and to grapple fervently with the "great matter of birth and death."

As I complete this manuscript, a pandemic rages throughout the world, authoritarianism has gained a new foothold in the West, and the climatic conditions on which all known human worlds have been built are under dire threat by the very humans who built them. In ancient China and India, spiritual seekers and officials in disfavor would go off to the forests or mountains to escape political chaos, seeking solitude in nature. Today, there is no escape to nature if the very configuration of nature that allows for human thriving is being undermined. Thus the Mahāyāna injunction to "save all sentient beings" today cannot but take on new and quite literal meanings, as entire species dwindle and disappear before our gaze. Meditative practices inevitably are worked into this salvific project and others of global import—to penetrate through the layered illusions of media, to find quite refuge amid the chaotic and frenzied demands of contemporary life, to nurture the monumental compassion necessary to "save all sentient beings." The practices we have been examining are among the many bequeathed to us by the dead and magnetically drawn to the world of the living, called forth by urgency as much as longing for quietude. And we shall see whether Iron-Age tools are able not only to bring personal calm but also to contribute to the transformation of the Anthropocene into a more livable age.

Notes

Chapter 1

1. https://www.lionsroar.com/remembering-sherab-zangmo-great-yogini-of-tibet/ (accessed December 19, 2020).
2. https://www.xrdc.org/events/meditation. See also: https://www.bbc.com/news/uk-engl and-london-46247339; https://www.dazeddigital.com/politics/article/48278/1/extinct ion-rebellion-staged-a-topless-protest-in-london-this-weekend; https://www.theguard ian.com/politics/2019/apr/01/wiggling-buttocks-enliven-existential-hell-of-brexit-deb ate; https://tricycle.org/trikedaily/extinction-rebellion-buddhists/ (all accessed December 19, 2020).
3. Nonomura (2009).
4. Perennial philosophy in this sense is the idea that all major philosophies and religions are different paths to the same goal. It was popularized in Aldous Huxley's *The Perennial Philosophy* (1945).
5. "Contemplation in Contexts: Tibetan Buddhist Meditation Across the Boundaries of the Humanities and Sciences." International Society for Contemplative Studies 2014 keynote address. https://www.youtube.com/watch?v=QEciEIaAUMM (accessed August 19, 2021).
6. In his book on the use of Buddhist meditation by psychotherapists, Ira Helderman uses the metaphor of filters to discuss what elements of Buddhism get filtered in the psychothera-peutic use of meditation. I adapting it more broadly, though, and apply it to a wide variety of cultural contexts in the modern world (Helderman 2019).
7. https://tergar.org/programs/what-is-the-joy-of-living/; https://learning.tergar.org/tag/ secular/ (accessed July 9, 2021).
8. I mean "liberalism" in this book not in the American sense of liberal-versus-conservative, but in the broader sense of the social and political philosophy dominant in much of the world espousing democracy, individual rights, freedom of choice, limited government, and free-market economics.
9. I will explain my particular use of this term later. For now, suffice to say it designates "the ways people imagine their social existence, how they fit together with others, how things go on between them and their fellows, the expectations that are normally met, and the deeper normative notions and images that underlie these expectations" (Taylor 2004, 23).
10. The ethic of health and well-being is, of course, amply addressed in the disciplines of psy-chology, neuroscience, and cognitive science. I am referring, however, to sociological, an-thropological, and religious studies perspectives that address their social and historical place. See Hickey (2019) for a historical investigation and evaluation of mindfulness as healthcare. For nuanced examinations of mindfulness as a social movement among elites in education, finance, business, etc., see Kucinskas (2019) and Chen (2022). For a more pointed critique of mindfulness in business culture, see Purser (2019).

Chapter 2

1. Buddhist Geeks Podcast, Episode 43, October 29, 2007. http://www.podcastsunited.com/Religion-and-Spirituality/Buddhism/Buddhist-Geeks.html?Page=32&Play=BG-043-Neuroscience-and-The-Enlightenment-Machine.
2. http://www.choosemuse.com.
3. https://www.accesstoinsight.org/lib/authors/soma/wayof.html (accessed July 14, 2021).
4. Patrick Stinson, "Overview of Vipassana Meditation." 2018. http://snowonthedesert.com/2018/03/overview-of-vipassana-meditation/ (accessed February 11, 2021).
5. American Mindfulness Research Association. https://goamra.org/resources/ (accessed June 22, 2020).
6. Some examples of such studies and a few books and articles discussing some of this research through the last couple decades include: Lutz, Dunne, and Davidson (2007); Hanson (2009); Rubia (2009); Grant et al. (2010); MacLean et al. (2010); Farb, Anderson, and Segal (2012); Tang et al. (2015); Goleman and Davidson (2017).
7. The phenomenological tradition offers alternative models, for example Heidegger's and Merleau-Ponty's nonrepresentational, enactive, and embodied analysis of human activity in relation to the world. Also see Lakoff and Johnson (1999); Noë (2010); and Taylor (2007, esp. 558–60), as well as many poststructuralist thinkers. For an alternative understanding of the role of emotions and perspective in knowing, see Martha Nussbaum (2001), who insists that emotion is essential to knowing and is itself a *kind* of knowing.
8. "Buddhism and Cognitive Science: How Can the Dialogue Move Forward?" Talk given at Buddhism, Mind, and Cognitive Science conference, University of California, Berkeley, April 25, 2014.
9. Some thinkers, in fact, argue that ordinary cognition is more like conversation or internal dialogue (Archer 2003). On this model, perhaps when this conversation is muted in certain meditative practices, consciousness *becomes*—rather than being discovered to be—granular, discrete, moment-to-moment thoughts. In this sense, an alternative model might be considered: mindfulness does, in fact, discover something—underlying processes that bubble up to create conscious narratives and internal dialogue—and, rather than perceiving them as objective truths, the meditator accesses some of the normally unconscious processes that feed into these aspects of consciousness that we normally inhabit and is able to shape them more intentionally or assess which dialogs to embrace and which to steer away from.
10. See, for example, Anderson (2014), Racine et al. (2005), Satel and Lilienfeld (2013).
11. On embodied cognition, see also Varela et al. (1991), Chemero (2009), Shapiro (2019).

Chapter 3

1. https://www.goldmansachs.com/careers/blog/posts/why-self-care-isnt-selfish.html (accessed August 10, 2021).
2. Sujato (2020, Kindle Locations 2441–2478).
3. For example, Samuel (2005), Mrozik (2007), Cook (2010), Collins (2018).
4. This is why I follow Steven Collins in translating *pratiques/technologies de soi* as "practices/technologies of self" rather than of "the self." The term, Collins insists, "is not referring to an abstract (philosophical) entity *the* self. . . . One could well translate the phrases as simply 'turning towards oneself,' or even, loosely, 'introspection.' They refer to a process, a project, a practice, and not to a metaphysic of 'the self' " (Collins 2018, 26).

5. This is a somewhat awkward translation of the French *imaginaire* that has, for better or worse, become common usage in English among social thinkers.
6. Lifeworld (Ger. *lebenswelt*) is in fact a similar concept developed in phenomenology, especially Husserl and Merleau-Ponty. It refers to the world not as a collection of objective facts, but the pretheoretical, subjective, and intersubjective experience of being in a world of things and people that all have particular meanings, significance, emotional valences. Husserl calls it the "ground" for all shared human experience in everyday life (Husserl, 1970 [1936], 142). It is, in short, the world as it exists *for us*. I distinguish it here from the social imaginary in that the latter extends the concept of the lifeworld somewhat to emphasize its intersubjective aspects and its tacit dimensions, as well as the role of imagination in constituting it.
7. For more on the concept of the social imaginary, see Taylor (2004). For a specific application to early Buddhism, see Collins (1998).

Chapter 4

1. Translation by Thanissaro Bhikkhu, https://www.accesstoinsight.org/tipitaka/kn/thag/thag.01.00x.than.html#passage-3 (accessed July 18, 2021).
2. Translation by K. R. Norman, https://www.accesstoinsight.org/tipitaka/kn/thag/thag.05.09.norm.html (accessed July 18, 2021).
3. What I am calling the "Pali Social Imaginary" masks a great deal of complexity and debate that would be inappropriate and unnecessary to address here. Suffice it to say that it is shorthand for the ideas, ideals, ethical stance, and general life-orientation that emerge from the Pali Canon (itself a contested term). Although this literature no doubt contains much that goes back to historically early Buddhism, it should not be uncritically assumed to represent "original Buddhism" or even "early Buddhism," since some parts of it are much later than others and, moreover, much of this literature was redacted nearly a millennium after the earliest iterations of Buddhist teachings. See Collins (1990) and Skilling et al. (2012).
4. This dominant culture is often characterized as Brahmanism. In Magadha, where the Buddha is said to have lived, however, Brahmanism may not have present by the time of the likely dates of the Buddha's life (Bronkhorst 2007). Certainly during the early solidification and development of Buddhist doctrine and practice, however, Brahmanism had become an important countervailing influence, and much of what gets recorded in the suttas certainly reflects that fact that Buddhist teaching often positioned itself in response to Brahmanism, whether or not that is true of the Buddha himself.
5. There is disagreement among scholars on just how central meditation was in Indian Buddhist monastic life. See, for example, Schopen (2004, 26ff.), Stuart (2015, vol. I, 18–26), Shulman (2014).
6. See, for example, M I 340, A I 25, S IV 301, and A II 164. Shaw (2006, 12–15) has a brief discussion of lay meditation in the Pali Canon and in Theravāda societies.
7. Translation by Maurice O'Connell Walshe, https://www.accesstoinsight.org/tipitaka/sn/sn03/sn03.013.wlsh.html (accessed July 30, 2021).
8. See Wynne (2007) and Bronkhorst (2000) for more on the early historical development of Buddhist meditation in the broader context of Indian ascetic movements.
9. For discussions of whether *sati* in its technical sense retains something of the sense of recollecting the past, as well as other nuances of the term, see Bodhi (2011), Dreyfus (2011).
10. There is also an expanded version, the *Great Sutta on the Foundations of Mindfulness* (*Mahāsatipaṭṭhhāna Sutta*, D 22, D ii 290) presents a complex and intriguing portrait of

meditation and its purposes in the South Asian Buddhist context. The two are essential the same except that the expanded version contains an extended discussion on the four noble truths and the eightfold path. There are a number of good translations of in print and online. For the shorter version, see Bodhi (1995, 145–55) and Soma Thera at http://www. accesstoinsight.org/tipitaka/mn/mn.010.soma.html. For the longer, see Walshe (1995) and Thanissaro Bhikkhu at http://www.accesstoinsight.org/tipitaka/dn/dn.22.0.than. html. There is some ambiguity in the title, which can be translated either as "setting up" or "establishing" (*upaṭṭhāna*) of mindfulness or "foundation" or "domain" (*paṭṭhāna*) of mindfulness. Thus, as Bhikkhu Bodhi says, "the four *satipaṭṭhānas* may be understood as either the four ways of setting up mindfulness or as the four objective domains of mindfulness" (Bodhi 1995, 1188–89).

11. This term is often translated "attention," but I am following Georges Dreyfus's helpful translation and interpretation (2011, 49).

12. For a comprehensive discussion of the terminology of meditation in the SP, see Anālayo (2003). See also, Bodhi (2011), Dreyfus (2011), Gethin (2011), Kuan (2008), Sujato (2005 [2012]).

13. Gunaratana (2002, 138).

14. How Heidegger could have been so incisive in his analysis of the "they-self" and apparently not seen more clearly its sinister operations in Nazi Germany is one of the great mysteries of philosophy (Trawny 2019)!

15. S 22.39; III 40. Translated by Thanissaro Bhikkhu, http://www.accesstoinsight.org/tipitaka/ sn/sn22/sn22.039.than.html (accessed January 14, 2013).

16. Translated by Thanissaro Bhikkhu, http://www.accesstoinsight.org/tipitaka/vin/sv/bhik khu-pati.html#sk-31 (accessed January 14, 2013).

Chapter 5

1. www.buddhanet.net/pdf_file/Sri-Lanka-monasteries.pdf (accessed February 4, 2010).

2. Translation by Thanissaro Bhikkhu, http://www.accesstoinsight.org/tipitaka/kn/snp/ snp.1.11.than.html (accessed March 21, 21).

3. Translation by Thanisarro Bhikkhu, https://www.accesstoinsight.org/tipitaka/kn/thag/ thag.02.16.than.html (accessed July 18, 2021).

4. The Sanskrit term *dharma* (Pali: *dhamma*) is one of the most polyvalent in the ancient Indian world. For our purposes, "Dharma"—with a capital D—refers to the teachings of the Buddha while *dharmas* refer to the basic constituents of experience or existence.

5. For a thoughtful account of how the SP does this, see Shulman (2014, ch. 3).

Chapter 6

1. Perhaps this more contextual conception of *experience* may help us recover a way of talking about experience in meditative practice in a way that avoids at least some of the problems elucidated by Robert Sharf in his influential article (1995). Meditative experience, as elucidated above, is not the bare empirical observation of mental contents, nor an isolated and private Cartesian perception mirroring reality but a dialogical process that is always in relation to the tradition and the broader culture, its categories, and ideals. It recognizes the rhetorical use and scholastic origins of much "experience language," yet also acknowledges the importance of interiority and self-reflexivity in the lives of meditators.

2. Wynne (2018) argues that there is a tension in the Pali literature between an approach in which "proper conditioning allows for a higher form of knowledge" and one in which "conditioning must be undone, 'consciousness' must be deconstructed" (96). In the following chapter, I pick up the latter approach as it is expressed in Mahāyāna literature, where it becomes more prominent.

Chapter 7

1. Ponlop (2020).
2. I adapted this idea from the Buddhist Studies scholar William Waldron, via Eyal Aviv.
3. For a detailed analysis of the Abhidharma of the Sarvāstivāda school, see Dhammjoti (2015).
4. For some further elaborations on the philosophy of emptiness in Perfection of Wisdom and Madhyamaka literature, see Lancaster, Gomez, and Conze (1977); Garfield (1995); McMahan (2002, ch 1); Walser (2005); Westerhoff (2009); Williams (2009), Siderits and Shōryū (2013).
5. For some in-depth discussions of various textual presentations of the doctrine of buddhanature, see Hookham (1991), King (1991), and Zimmerman (2002).

Chapter 8

1. https://www.headspace.com/articles/how-to-be-more-grateful (accessed August 12, 2021).
2. The "10,000 rule" was popularized by Malcolm Gladwell in his book *Outliers*. It claims that as a general rule it takes 10,000 hours to master a complex skill like playing a musical instrument (and has since been criticized). Meditation researchers have applied the rule to determining whether a person should be considered an advanced meditator for research purposes.
3. See, for example, Batchelor (2010, 2015) and the Secular Buddhism website: https://secularbuddhism.com/.
4. There is an argument to be made for a kind of secularism in the ancient world as well (see https://www.multiple-secularities.de/media/multiple_secularities_research_programme.pdf), but I am referring here specifically to modern, post-Enlightenment versions.
5. For a comparative analysis of how different configurations of secularism in the United States, China, and India have shaped the practice of meditation and the possibilities for the practice of Buddhism, see McMahan (2017).
6. For Kabat-Zinn's own account of how he and others developed MBSR, see Kabat-Zinn (2011). For a critique of such programs in public schools that illustrates the stakes of the designation of mindfulness practices as "religious" or "secular," see Brown (2019).
7. John Lardas Modern (2011) discusses this pervasive, "spectral" aspect of secularism in the American context.
8. http://www.fodian.net/world/0217.html (accessed April 29, 2020).
9. For a more complete version see Smith (1991).
10. From the *Caṇḍamahāroṣaṇa Tantra* 10.20–10.22. Toh 431 Degé Kangyur, vol. 80 (rgyud 'bum, nga), folios 304.b–343.a. Translated by the Dharmachakra Translation Committee under the patronage and supervision of 84000: Translating the Words of the Buddha. https://read.84000.co/translation/toh431.html (accessed January 29, 2021).

Chapter 9

1. https://insighttimer.com/meditation-topics/authenticity.
2. https://www.huffpost.com/entry/brene-brown-how-to-be-yourself_n_5786554.
3. For more extensive examination of the ideal of authenticity, see Ferrara (1993); Taylor (1991, 1989), Varga (2011), Varga and Guignon (2020).
4. For samples of this type of critique, see Carrette and King (2005), Purser (2019).

Chapter 10

1. Translated from the Pali by Thanissaro Bhikkhu. https://www.accesstoinsight.org/tipitaka/kn/thig/thig.01.00x.than.html (accessed June 7, 2021)
2. Vassakāra translation. https://www.accesstoinsight.org/tipitaka/an/an04/an04.035.than.html#fn-1
3. In addition to Verchery's work, I am indebted to Mengxiao Wu for helping me gain some understanding of this community.

Chapter 11

1. I say "sense of human agency" in that I am not making an argument about the philosophical question of free will but sticking to the phenomenology of meditative experience. For a fuller philosophical exploration of free will, mental causation, and mental freedom in relation to meditation, see Repetti (2019).
2. Some books, both scholarly and popular, developing this idea include: Yancy and McRae (2019), Magee (2019), Yetunde and Giles (2020).
3. https://www.buddhistinquiry.org/course/what-gets-left-out-expanding-practice-community-and-freedom/ (accessed June 22,2020).
4. https://calendar.spiritrock.org/events/white-and-awakening-together-2020/ (accessed August 1, 2020).
5. https://oneearthsangha.org/programs/2019-ecosattva-training/ (accessed August 14, 2020).
6. Dr. Sophie Botros and Sergei Abramov, in a letter to *The Guardian* in response to Ron Purser's article "The Mindfulness Conspiracy." https://www.theguardian.com/lifeandstyle/2019/jun/16/mindfulness-can-be-an-active-force-for-change-in-the-world.

Chapter 12

1. See, for example, Jason Ananda Josephson-Storm's critique of the "myth of disenchantment" (2017).
2. Michael Venables, "Review: Yayoi Kusama: Infinity Mirrors—Of Dots and Emptiness." https://medium.com/future-technology-and-society/review-yayoi-kusama-infinity-mirrors-dots-and-a-sense-of-emptiness-f6ebf8bf363e (accessed January 5, 2019).
3. For an extended version of this story, see McMahan 2008, chapter 6.

Works Cited

Abi-Rached, Joelle, and Nikolas Rose. "The Birth of the Neuromolecular Gaze." *History of the Human Sciences* 23, no. 1 (2010): 11–36.

Addiss, Stephen, Stanley Lombardo, and Judith Roitman. *Zen Sourcebook: Traditional Documents from China, Korea, and Japan*. Indianapolis: Hackett, 2008.

Anālayo. *Satipaṭṭhāna: The Direct Path to Realization*. Birmingham: Windhorse, 2003.

Anderson, Ellen, Cynthia Willett, and Diana Meyers. "Feminist Perspectives on the Self." *The Stanford Encyclopedia of Philosophy* (Spring 2020 Edition), Edward N. Zalta (ed.), https://plato.stanford.edu/archives/spr2020/entries/feminism-self/.

Anderson, Michael L. *After Phrenology: Neural Reuse and the Interactive Brain*. Boston: MIT Press, 2014.

Archer, Margaret. *Structure, Agency, and the Internal Conversation*. Cambridge: Cambridge University Press, 2003.

Arntzen, Sonja. *Ikkyu and the Crazy Cloud Anthology*. Tokyo: University of Tokyo Press, 1987.

Asad, Talal. *Formations of the Secular: Christianity, Islam, Modernity*. Palo Alto: Stanford University Press, 2003.

Aviv, Rachel. "The Unraveling of a Dancer." *The New Yorker*. April 6, 2020.

Barrett, Lisa Feldman. *How Emotions Are Made: The Secret Life of the Brain*. Boston: Houghton Mifflin Harcourt, 2017.

Barrett, William. "Zen for the West." In Daisetz T. Suzuki, *Essays in Zen Buddhism*, xii–xx. New York: Grove Weidenfeld, 1961.

Batchelor, Stephen. *After Buddhism: Rethinking the Dharma for a Secular Age*. New Haven: Yale University Press, 2015.

Batchelor, Stephen. *Confession of a Buddhist Atheist*. New York: Spiegel & Grau, 2010.

Baumann, Zygmunt. *Liquid Life*. Cambridge, UK: Polity Press, 2005.

Bellah, Robert, Richard Madsen, William Sullivan, Ann Swidler, and Steven M. Tipton. *Habits of the Heart: Individualism and Commitment in American Life*. Berkeley: University of California Press, 1985.

Bielefeldt, Carl. *Dōgen's Manuals of Zen Meditation*. Berkeley: University of California Press, 1988.

Bishop, Scott R., Mark Lau, Shauna Shapiro, Linda Carlson, Nicole D. Anderson, James Carmody, Zindel V. Segal, et al. "Mindfulness: A Proposed Definition." *Clinical Psychology: Science and Practice* 11 (2004): 230–41.

Bodhi, Bhikkhu, trans. *The Connected Discourses of the Buddha: A Translation of the Saṃyutta Nikāya*. 2nd ed. Boston: Wisdom Publications, 2000.

Bodhi, Bhikkhu, trans. *The Middle Length Discourses of the Buddha: A New Translation of the Majjhima Nikāya*. Boston: Wisdom Publications, 1995.

Bodhi, Bhikkhu. "What Does Mindfulness Really Mean? A Canonical Perspective." *Contemporary Buddhism: An Interdisciplinary Journal* 12 (2011): 19–39.

Bodhidharma. *The Zen Teaching of Bodhidharma*. Translated by Red Pine. New York: North Point Press, 1987.

Borup, Jørn. *Japanese Rinzai Zen Buddhism*. Leiden and Boston: Brill, 2008.

Bourdieu, Pierre. *Outline of a Theory of Practice*. Cambridge: Cambridge University Press, 1977.

Braun, Erik. *The Birth of Insight: Meditation, Modern Buddhism, and the Burmese Monk Ledi Sayadaw*. Chicago: University of Chicago Press, 2013.

Breckenridge, Carol Appadurai, and Peter van der Veer. "Orientalism and the Postcolonial Predicament." In Carol Appadurai Breckenridge and Peter van der Veer, eds. *Orientalism and the Postcolonial Predicament: Perspectives on South Asia*, 1–19. Philadelphia: University of Pennsylvania Press, 1993.

Bronkhorst, Johannes. *The Two Traditions of Meditation in Ancient India*. Delhi: Motilal Banarsidas, 2000 [1993].

Bronkhorst, Johannes. *Greater Magadha: Studies in the Culture of Early India*. Leiden: Brill, 2007.

Brown, Candy Gunther. *Debating Yoga and Mindfulness in Public Schools Reforming Secular Education or Reestablishing Religion?* Chapel Hill: University of North Carolina Press, 2019.

Butler, Judith. *Senses of the Subject*. New York: Fordham University Press, 2015.

Carrette, J., and Richard King. *Selling Spirituality: The Silent Takeover of Religion*. London and New York: Routledge, 2005.

Carus, Paul. *The Gospel of Buddhism, Compiled from Ancient Records*. Chicago and London: Open Court, 1915.

Cassiniti, Julia. "Wherever You Go, There You Aren't? Non-Self, Spirits, and the Concept of the Person in Thai Buddhist Mindfulness." In David L. McMahan and Erik Braun, eds. *Meditation, Buddhism, and Science*, 133–50. New York: Oxford University Press, 2017.

Chemero, Anthony. *Radical Embodied Cognitive Science*. Cambridge, MA: MIT Press, 2009.

Chen, Carolyn. *Work Pray Code: When Work Becomes Religion in Silicon Valley*. Princeton: Princeton University Press, 2022.

Clark, Simone. *Mindful Eating for Lasting Weight-Loss: Surround Yourself with Mindful Moments for Long-Term Sustainable Weight Loss*. Independently published, 2020.

Cleary, Thomas F., trans. *Entry into the Realm of Reality: The Text*. Boulder, CO: Shambhala, 1989.

Cleary, Thomas F, trans. *Zen Essence: The Science of Freedom*. Boston: Shambhala, 1989.

Clough, Bradly S. *Early Indian and Theravada Buddhism: Soteriological Controversy and Diversity*. Amherst: Cambria, 2012.

Collins, Steven. "Hadot, Foucault, and Comparison with Buddhism." In David V. Fiordalis, ed. *Buddhist Spiritual Practices: Thinking with Pierre Hadot on Buddhism, Philosophy, and the Path*, 21–59. Berkeley: Mangalam Press, 2018.

Collins, Steven. *Nirvana and Other Buddhist Felicities: Utopias of the Pali Imaginaire*. New York: Cambridge University Press, 1998.

Collins, Steven. "On the Very Idea of the Pali Canon." *Journal of the Pali Text Society* 15 (1990): 89–126.

Conze, Edward. *The Perfection of Wisdom in Eight Thousand Lines and Its Verse Summary*. San Francisco: Four Seasons Foundation, 1973.

Conze, Edward, trans. *The Large Sutra on Perfect Wisdom: With the Divisions of the Abhisamayālaṅkāra*. Berkeley: University of California Press, 1975.

Cook, Joanna. *Meditation in Modern Buddhism: Renunciation and Change in Thai Monastic Life*. Cambridge: Cambridge University Press, 2010.

Cook, Joanna. "'Mind the Gap': Appearance and Reality in Mindfulness-Based Cognitive Therapy." In David L. McMahan and Erik Braun, eds. *Meditation, Buddhism, and Science*, 144–32. New York: Oxford University Press, 2017.

Crawford, Matthew B. *The World beyond Your Head: On Becoming an Individual in an Age of Distraction*. New York: Farrar, Straus & Giroux, 2015.

Crosby, Kate. *Traditional Theravāda Meditation and Its Modern-Era Suppression*. Hong Kong: Buddhist Dharma Centre of Hong Kong, 2013.

Dalai Lama, the Fourteenth. *Beyond Religion: Ethics for the Whole World*. New York: Houghton Mifflin Harcourt, 2011.

Dhammjoti, Bhikkhu K. L. *Sarvāstivāda Abhidharma*. Hong Kong: The Buddha-Dharma Centre of Hong Kong 2015 [2002].

Dharmapala, Anagarika. *Return to Righteousness: A Collection of Speeches, Essays and Letters of the Anagarika Dharmapala*. Ceylon: Government Press, 1965.

Dreyfus, Georges B. J. "Is Mindfulness Present-Centered and Non-Judgmental? A Discussion of the Cognitive Dimensions of Mindfulness." *Contemporary Buddhism: An Interdisciplinary Journal* 12, no. 1 (2011): 41–54.

Dreyfus, H. L. *Being-in-the-World: A Commentary on Heidegger's Being and Time, Division I*. Cambridge, MA: MIT Press, 1990.

Dunne, John D. "Toward an Understanding of Nondual Mindfulness." *Contemporary Buddhism: An Interdisciplinary Journal* 12, no. 1 (2011): 71–88.

Dunne, John D. "Buddhist Styles of Mindfulness: A Heuristic Approach." In Brian D. Ostafin, Michael D. Robinson, and Brian P. Meier, eds. *Handbook of Mindfulness and Self-Regulation*, 251–70. New York: Springer, 2015.

Embree, Ainslie T. *Sources of Indian Tradition: Volume One: From the Beginning to 1800*. 2nd ed. New York: Columbia University Press, 1988 [1958].

Farb, Norman A. S., Adam K. Anderson, and Zindel V. Segal. "The Mindful Brain and Emotion Regulation in Mood Disorders." *Canadian Journal of Psychiatry* 57, no. 2 (2012): 70–77.

Ferrara, Alessandro, *Modernity and Authenticity: A Study of the Social and Ethical Thought of Jean-Jacques Rousseau*. Albany: SUNY Press, 1993.

Fiordalis, David V. ed. *Buddhist Spiritual Practices: Thinking with Pierre Hadot on Buddhism, Philosophy, and the Path*. Berkeley: Mangalam Press, 2018.

Forman, Robert K. ed. *The Problem of Pure Consciousness: Mysticism and Philosophy*. New York: Oxford University Press, 1990.

Foucault, Michel. *Essential Works of Michel Foucault*, Vol. 1: *Ethics: Subjectivity and Truth*. Edited by P. Rabinow. London: Allen Lane, 2000.

Foucault, Michel. *The History of Sexuality*, Vol. 2: *The Use of Pleasure*. New York: Pantheon Books, 1978.

Fromm, Erich. *Zen Buddhism and Psychoanalysis*. New York: Grove Press, 1960.

Garfield, Jay. *The Fundamental Wisdom of the Middle Way: Nāgārjuna's Mūlamadhyamakakāri kā*. New York: Oxford University Press, 1995.

Gaus, Gerald, Shane D. Courtland, and David Schmidtz. "Liberalism." *The Stanford Encyclopedia of Philosophy* (Fall 2020 Edition), Edward N. Zalta (ed.), https://plato.stanford.edu/archives/fall2020/entries/liberalism/.

Gergen, Kenneth. *The Saturated Self: Dilemmas of Identity in Contemporary Life*. New York: Basic Books, 2000 [1990].

Gethin, Rupert. "On Some Definitions of Mindfulness." *Contemporary Buddhism: An Interdisciplinary Journal* 12, no. 1 (2011): 263–79.

Giddens, Anthony. *Modernity and Self-Identity. Self and Society in the Late Modern Age*. Cambridge: Polity Press, 1991.

Gibson, James J. *The Ecological Approach to Visual Perception*. Boston: Houghton Mifflin Harcourt, 1979.

Gleig, Ann. *American Dharma: Buddhism beyond Modernity*. New Haven: Yale University Press, 2019.

Goenka, S. N. *Meditation Now: Inner Peace through Inner Wisdom*. Onalaska: Vipassana Research Institute, 2002.

Goleman, Daniel, and Richard Davidson. *The Science of Meditation: How to Change Your Brain, Mind and Body*. New York: Penguin, 2017.

Golomb, Jacob. *In Search of Authenticity from Kierkegaard to Camus*. London and New York: Routledge, 1995.

Govinda, Anagarika. *Creative Meditation and Multi-Dimensional Consciousness*. Wheaton, IL: Theosophical Publishing House, 1976.

Goyal, M, S. Singh, E. M. S. Sibinga, N. F. Gould, A. Rowland-Seymour, R. Sharma, Z. Berger, et al. "Meditation Programs for Psychological Stress and Well-Being: A Systematic Review and Meta-Analysis." *Journal of the American Medical Association, Internal Medicine* 174, no. 3 (2014): 357–68.

Grant, J. A., J. Courtemanche, G. H. Duncan, and P. Rainville. "Cortical Thickness and Pain Sensitivity in Zen Meditators." *Emotion* 10, no. 1 (2010): 43–53.

Green, Thomas Hill. *Lectures on the Principles of Political Obligation and Other Essays*. Edited by Paul Harris and John Morrow. Cambridge: Cambridge University Press, 1986 [1895].

Grosnick, William H. "The *Tathāgathgarbha Sūtra*." In Donald S. Lopez, ed. *Buddhism in Practice*, 92–106. Princeton: Princeton University Press, 1995.

Guignon, Charles. *On Being Authentic*. London: Routledge, 2004.

Gunaratana, Henepola. *Mindfulness in Plain English*. Boston: Wisdom Publications, 2002 [1993].

Hanson, Rick. *Buddha's Brain*. With Richard Mendius. Oakland, CA: New Harbinger Publications, 2009.

Harris, Sam. *Waking Up: A Guide to Spirituality without Religion*. New York: Simon & Schuster, 2014.

Hatchell, Christopher. *Naked Seeing: The Great Perfection, the Wheel of Time, and Visionary Buddhism in Renaissance Tibet*. New York: Oxford University Press, 2014.

Heidegger, Martin. *Being and Time*. Translated by John Macquarrie and Edward Robinson. New York: Harper & Row, 1962 [1927].

Heim, Maria. "Four Some Analyses of Feeling." In Maria Heim, Chakravarthi Ram-Prasad, and Roy Tzohar, eds. *The Bloomsbury Research Handbook of Emotions in Classical Indian Philosophy*, 87–106. London and New York: Bloomsbury Academic, 2021.

Heine, Steven, and Dale S. Wright, eds. *Zen Ritual: Studies of Zen Theory in Practice*. New York: Oxford University Press, 2007.

Helderman, Ira. *Prescribing the Dharma: Psychotherapists, Buddhist Traditions, and Defining Religion*. Chapel Hill: University of North Carolina Press, 2019.

Heuman, Linda. "Don't Believe the Hype." *Tricycle: The Buddhist Review*, October 1, 2014. https://tricycle.org/article/dont-believe-hype/.

Hickey, Wakoh Shannon. *Mind Cure: How Meditation Became Medicine*. New York: Oxford University Press, 2019.

Hookham, S. K. *The Buddha Within: Tathagatagarbha Doctrine According to the Shentong Interpretation of the Ratnagotravibhaga*. Suny Series in Buddhist Studies. Albany: SUNY Press, 1991.

Hsu, Funie. "American Cultural Baggage: The Racialized Secularization of Mindfulness in Schools." In Richard Payne, ed. *Secularizing Buddhism: New Perspectives on a Dynamic Tradition*, 79–93. Boston: Shambhala, 2021.

Humphries, Christmas, ed. *The Wisdom of Buddhism*. Abingdon: Curzon Press, 1987.

Husserl, Edmund. *The Crisis of European Sciences and Transcendental Phenomenology: An Introduction to Phenomenological Philosophy*. Translated by David Carr. Northwestern University Studies in Phenomenology & Existential Philosophy. Evanston: Northwestern University Press, 1970.

Huxley, Aldous. *The Perennial Philosophy*. New York: Harper, 1970 [1945].

Iwamura, Jane Naomi. *Virtual Orientalism: Asian Religions and American Popular Culture*. Oxford and New York: Oxford University Press, 2011.

Jamgon Kongtrul. *Jamgon Kongtrul's Retreat Manual*. Translated by Ngawang Zangpo. Ithaca: Snow Lion Press, 1994.

Jay, Martin. "A History of Alienation." *Aeon*. March 14, 2018. https://aeon.co/essays/in-the-1950s-everybody-cool-was-a-little-alienated-what-changed.

Jerryson, Michael, and Mark Juergensmeyer. *Buddhist Warfare*. New York and Oxford: Oxford University Press, 2010.

Kabat-Zinn, Jon. *Full Catastrophe Living: Using the Wisdom of Your Body and Mind to Face Stress, Pain, and Illness*. New York: Bantam, 2013 [1990].

Kabat-Zinn, Jon. "Some Reflections on the Origins of MBSR, Skilfull Means, and the Trouble with Maps." *Contemporary Buddhism: An Interdisciplinary Journal* 12, no. 1 (2011): 281–306.

Kabat-Zinn, Jon. *Wherever You Go, There You Are: Mindfulness Meditation in Everyday Life*. New York: Hyperion, 1994.

Kahn, Jonathon Samuel, and Vincent W. Lloyd, eds. *Race and Secularism in America*. Religion, Culture, and Public Life. New York: Columbia University Press, 2016.

Kahneman, Daniel. *Thinking, Fast and Slow*. New York: Farrar, Straus and Giroux, 2011.

Katz, Steven. *Mysticism and Philosophical Analysis*. New York: Oxford University Press, 1978.

Kaza, Stephanie. *Green Buddhism: Practice and Compassionate Action in Uncertain Times*. Boulder, CO: Shambhala, 2019.

Keane, Webb. *Ethical Life: Its Natural and Social Histories*. Princeton, NJ: Princeton University Press, 2015.

King, Richard. *Orientalism and Religion: Postcolonial Theory, India and the "Mystic East."* London and New York: Routledge, 1999.

King, Sallie. *Buddha Nature*. Albany: State University of New York Press, 1991.

Kirmayer, Lawrence J. "Mindfulness in Cultural Context." *Transcultural Psychiatry* 52, no. 4 (2015): 447–69.

Konnikova, Maria. "The Power of Concentration." *New York Times*. December 15, Section SR, p. 8, 2012.

Kopp, Sheldon. *If You Meet the Buddha on the Road, Kill Him! The Pilgrimage of Psychotherapy Patients*. New York: Bantam, 1976 [1972].

Kornfield, Jack. *After the Ecstasy, the Laundry: How the Heart Grows Wise on the Spiritual Path*. New York: Bantam Books, 2000.

Kuan, Tse-fu. *Mindfulness in Early Buddhism: New Approaches through Psychology and Textual Analysis of Pali, Chinese and Sanskrit Sources*. Abingdon: Routledge, 2008.

Kucinskas, Jaime. *The Mindful Elite: Mobilizing from the Inside Out*. New York: Oxford University Press, 2019.

LaFleur, William. "Enlightenment for Plants and Trees." In Mary Evelyn Tucker and Duncan Ryūkan Williams, eds. *Buddhism and Ecology: The Interconnection of Dharma and Deeds*, 109–16. Cambridge, MA: Harvard University Center for the Study of World Religions Publications, 1998.

Laidlaw, James. *The Subject of Virtue: An Anthropology of Ethics and Freedom*. New Departures in Anthropology. New York: Cambridge University Press, 2014.

Lakoff, George, and Mark Johnson. *Philosophy in the Flesh: The Embodied Mind and Its Challenge to Western Thought*. New York: Basic Books, 1999.

Lancaster, Lewis, Luis O. Gómez, Edward Conze, eds. *Prajñāpāramitā and Related Systems: Studies in Honor of Edward Conze*. Berkeley: University of California Press, 1977.

Latour, Bruno. *We Have Never Been Modern*. Translated by Catherine Porter. Cambridge, MA: Harvard University Press, 1993.

Lasch, Christopher. *The Culture of Narcissism: American Life in an Age of Diminishing Expectations*. New York: W. W. Norton, Inc., 1991 [1979].

Leighton, Dan. "Zen as Enactment Ritual." In Steven Heine and Dale S. Wright, eds. *Zen Ritual: Studies of Zen Theory in Practice*, 167–83. New York: Oxford University Press, 2007.

Lindahl, Jared R., and Willoughby B. Britton. "'I Have This Feeling of Not Really Being Here': Buddhist Meditation and Changes in Sense of Self." *Journal of Consciousness Studies* 26, no. 7–8 (2019): 157–83.

Lopez, Donald S. *Buddhism & Science: A Guide for the Perplexed.* Chicago: University of Chicago Press, 2008.

Lopez, Donald S. *The Scientific Buddha: His Short and Happy Life.* The Terry Lectures. New Haven, CT: Yale University Press, 2012.

Loy, David. *Ecodharma: Buddhist Teachings for the Ecological Crisis.* Somerville, MA: Wisdom Publications, 2019.

Luhrmann, T. M. *How God Becomes Real: Kindling the Presence of Invisible Others.* Princeton, NJ: Princeton University Press, 2020.

Luhrmann, T. M. *When God Talks Back: Understanding the American Evangelical Relationship with God.* New York: Alfred A. Knopf, 2012.

Lutz, Antoine, John Dunne, and Richard J. Davidson. "Meditation and the Neuroscience of Consciousness: An Introduction." In E. Thompson, M. Moscovitch, and P.D. Zelazo, eds. *Cambridge Handbook of Consciousness,* 499–553. Cambridge: Cambridge University Press, 2007.

MacLean, Katherine A., Emilio Ferrer, Stephen R. Aichele, David A. Bridwell, Anthony P. Zanesco, Tonya L. Jacobs, Brandon G. King, et al. "Intensive Meditation Training Improves Perceptual Discrimination and Sustained Attention." *Psychological Science* 21 (2010): 829–39.

MacPherson, C. B. *The Political Theory of Possessive Individualism.* Oxford: Oxford University Press, 1962.

Macy, Joanna. *World as Lover; World as Self.* Berkeley: Parallax Press, 1991.

Maezumi, Taishan, Roshi. *Appreciate Your Life: The Essence of Zen Practice.* Boston and London: Shambhala, 2002.

Magee, Rhonda V. *The Inner Work of Racial Justice: Healing Ourselves and Transforming Our Communities through Mindfulness.* New York: TarcherPerigee, 2019.

Mahmood, Saba. "Feminist Theory, Embodiment, and the Docile Agent: Some Reflections on the Egyptian Islamic Revival." *Cultural Anthropology* 16, no. 2 (May 2001): 202–36.

Mahmood, Saba. *Politics of Peity: The Islamic Revival and the Feminist Subject.* Princeton, NJ: Princeton University Press, 2005.

Makari, George. *The Soul Machine: The Invention of the Modern Mind.* New York: Norton, 2015.

Mariotti, Shanon. "Zen and the Art of Democracy: Contemplative Practice as Ordinary Political Theory." *Political Theory* 48, no. 4 (2020): 469–95.

McClelland, Tom. "The Mental Affordance Hypothesis." *Mind* 129, no. 514 (April 2020): 401–27.

McMahan, David. "Buddhism, Meditation, and Global Secularisms." *Journal of Global Buddhism* 18 (2017): 122–28.

McMahan, David L. *Empty Vision: Metaphor and Visionary Imagery in Mahâyâna Buddhism.* New York and London: RoutledgeCurzon, 2002.

McMahan, David L. "The Enchanted Secular: Buddhism and the Emergence of Transtraditional 'Spirituality.'" *Eastern Buddhist* 43, no. 1–2 (2012): 205–23.

McMahan, David L. *The Making of Buddhist Modernism.* New York: Oxford University Press, 2008.

McMahan, David, and Erik Braun, eds. *Meditation, Buddhism, and Science.* New York: Oxford University Press, 2017.

McRae, John R., trans. "Essentials of the Transmission of Mind." In *Zen Texts,* 3–43. BDK English Tripiṭaka Series. Berkeley: Numata Center for Buddhist Translation and Research, 2005.

McRae, John R., trans. *The Platform Sutra of the Sixth Patriarch.* BDK English Tripiṭaka Series. Berkeley: Numata Center for Buddhist Translation and Research, 2000.

Metzinger, Thomas. "The Problem of Mental Action." *Philosophy and Predictive Action* (2017). https://predictive-mind.net/papers/the-problem-of-mental-action.

Meyers, Diana T. *Subjection and Subjectivity*. New York: Routledge, 1994.

Mitra, Rejendralal, ed. *Aṣṭasāhasrikā Prajñāpāramitā*. Calcutta: Bibliotheca Indica, 1888.

Modern, John Lardas. *Secularism in Antebellum America*. Chicago: University of Chicago Press, 2011.

Mrozik, Susanne. *Virtuous Bodies: The Physical Dimensions of Morality in Buddhist Ethics*. New York: Oxford University Press, 2007.

Ñāṇamoli, Bhikkhu, trans. *The Middle Length Discourses of the Buddha: A New Translation of the Majjhima Nikāya*. Boston: Wisdom Publications, 1995.

Ñāṇamoli, Bhikkhu, trans. *The Path of Purification (Visuddhimagga)* by Buddhaghosa. Berkeley: Shambhala 1976 [1956].

Nelson, Maggie. *On Freedom: Four Songs of Care and Constraint*. Minneapolis: Graywolf Press, 2021.

Newberg, Andrew, and Mark Robert Waldman. *How Enlightenment Changes Your Brain: The New Science of Transformation*. New York: Avery Press, 2016.

Nhat Hanh, Thich. *The Heart of Understanding: Commentaries on the Prajñaparamita Heart Sutra*. Berkeley, CA: Parallax Press, 1988.

Nhat Hanh, Thich. *Peace Is Every Step: The Path of Mindfulness in Everyday Life*. New York: Bantam, 1991.

Noë, Alvin. *Out of Our Heads: Why You Are Not Your Brain, and Other Lessons from the Biology of Consciousness*. New York: Macmillan, 2010.

Nonomura, Kaoru. *Eat Sleep Sit: My Year at Japan's Most Rigorous Zen Temple*. Translated by Juliet Winters Carpenter. Tokyo/New York: Kodansha International, 2009.

Nussbaum, Martha. *Upheavals of Thought: the Intelligence of Emotions*. Cambridge: Cambridge University Press, 2001.

Nyanaponika Thera. *The Heart of Buddhist Meditation*. Kandy: Buddhist Meditation Society, 1954.

Olivelle, Patrick. "Ascetic Withdrawal or Social Engagement." In Donald S. Lopez, ed. *Religions of India in Practice*, 543–45. Princeton Readings in Religions. Princeton, NJ: Princeton University Press, 1995.

Ospina, Maria B., et al. "Meditation Practices for Health: State of the Research." Evidence Report/Technology Assessment No. 155. AHRQ Publication No. 07-E010. Rockville, MD: Agency for Healthcare Research and Quality, 2007.

Pagis, Michal. *Inward: Vipassana Meditation and the Embodiment of the Self*. Chicago: University of Chicago Press, 2019.

Payne, Richard, ed. *Secularizing Buddhism: New Perspectives on a Dynamic Tradition*. Boston: Shambhala, 2021.

Ponlop, Rinpoche. "How to Do Mahamudra Meditation." *Lion's Roar*. November 2020. https://www.lionsroar.com/how-to-meditate-dzogchen-ponlop-rinpoche-on-mahamudra/.

Purser, Ronald E. *McMindfulness: How Mindfulness Became the New Capitalist Spirituality*. London: Repeater, 2019.

Putnam, Robert. *Bowling Alone: The Collapse and Revival of American Community*. New York: Simon & Schuster, 2000.

Racine, E., Bar-Ilan, O., & Illes, J. "fMRI in the Public Eye." *Nature Reviews Neuroscience* 6 (2005): 159–64.

Ramstead, M. J., S. P. Veissière, and L. J. Kirmayer. "Cultural Affordances: Scaffolding Local Worlds through Shared Intentionality and Regimes of Attention." *Frontiers in Psychology* 7 (2016). https://doi.org/10.3389/fpsyg.2016.01090.

Repetti, Rick. *Buddhism, Meditation, and Free Will: A Theory of Mental Freedom*. Abingdon and New York: Routledge Press, 2019.

Reps, Paul. *Zen Flesh, Zen Bones*. Tokyo: C.E. Tuttle, 1957.

Ricard, Matthieu. *On the Path to Enlightenment: Heart Advice from Great Tibetan Masters*. Boston: Shambhala Publications, 2013.

Richard Rorty. *Philosophy and the Mirror of Nature*. Princeton, NJ: Princeton University Press, 1979.

Rose, Nikolas. "The Neurochemical Self and Its Anomalies." In Aaron Doyle and Richard Ericson, eds. *Risk and Morality*, 407–37. Toronto: University of Toronto Press, 2003.

Rose, Nikolas, and Joelle M. Abi-Rached. *Neuro: The New Brain Sciences and the Management of the Mind*. Princeton, NJ: Princeton University Press, 2013.

Rousseau, Jean-Jacques. "On the Social Contract." In Mitchell Cohen and Nicole Fermon, eds. *Princeton Readings in Political Thought*, 280–92. Princeton, NJ: Princeton University Press, 1996.

Rubia, K. "The Neurobiology of Meditation and Its Clinical Effectiveness in Psychiatric Disorders." *Biological Psychology* 82 (2009): 1–11.

Rutschman-Byler, Jiryu Mark. *Two Shores of Zen: An American Monk's Japan*. Lulu.com, 2009.

Samuel, Geoffrey. *Tantric Revisionings: New Understandings of Tibetan Buddhism and Indian Religion*. Aldershot; Burlington, VT: Ashgate, 2005.

Satel, Sally, and Scott O. Lilienfeld. *Brainwashed: The Seductive Appeal of Mindless Neuroscience*. New York: Basic Books, 2013.

Sartre, Jean-Paul. *Being and Nothingness: A Phenomenological Essay on Ontology*. New York: Washington Square Press, 1992 [1943].

Schopen, Gregory. "The Monastic Ownership of Servants or Slaves: Local and Legal Factors in the Redactional History of Two Vinayas." *Journal of the International Association of Buddhist Studies* 17, no. 2 (Winter 1994): 145–74.

Schopen, Gregory. *Buddhist Monks and Business Matters: Still More Papers on Monastic Buddhism in India*. Honolulu: University of Hawaii Press, 2004.

Senzaki, Nyōgen. *101 Zen Stories*. Philadelphia: David McKay Co., 1919.

Shapiro, Lawrence A. *Embodied Cognition*. New York: Routledge, 2019.

Sharf, Robert H. "Buddhist Modernism and the Rhetoric of Meditative Experience." *Numen* 42, no. 3 (1995): 228–83.

Sharf, Robert H. "Visualization and Mandala in Shingon Buddhism." In Robert H. Sharf and Elizabeth Horton Sharf, eds. *Living Images*, 151–98. Stanford: Stanford University Press, 2001.

Shaw, Sarah. *Buddhist Meditation: An Anthology of Texts from the Pāli Canon*. London and New York: Routledge, 2006.

Shils, Edward. *Tradition*. Chicago: University of Chicago Press, 1981.

Shorter, Edward. *From Paralysis to Fatigue: A History of Psychosomatic Illness in the Modern Era*. New York: Free Press, 1992.

Shulman, Eviatar. "Mindful Wisdom: The Sati-paṭṭhāna-sutta on Mindfulness, Memory, and Liberation." *History of Religions* 49, no. 4 (2010): 393–420.

Shulman, Eviatar. *Rethinking the Buddha*. Cambridge: Cambridge University Press, 2014.

Siderits, Mark, and Katsura Shōryū, trans. *Nāgārjuna. Nāgārjuna's Middle Way: Mūlamadhyamakākarikā*. Classics of Indian Buddhism. Boston: Wisdom Publications, 2013.

Skilling, Peter, Jason A. Carbine, Claudio Cicuzza, and Santi Pakdeekham, eds. *How Theravāda Is Theravāda? Exploring Buddhist Identities*. Chiang Mai: Silkworm Books, 2012.

Smith, Caleb. "Disciplines of Attention in a Secular Age." *Critical Inquiry* 45, no. 4 (2019): 884–909.

Smith, Wilfred Cantwell. *The Meaning and End of Religion*. Minneapolis: Fortress Press, 1991.

Sōen (Soyen) Shaku. *Zen for Americans: Including the Sutra of Forty-Two Chapters*. New York: Barnes and Noble Books, 1993 [1913].

Stanley, Steven. "Mindfulness: Toward a Critical-Relational Perspective." *Social and Personality Psychology Compass* 6, no. 9 (2012): 631–41.

Stuart, Daniel M. *A Less Traveled Path: Saddharmasmṛtyupasthānasūtra chapter 2*. 2 vols. Beijing and Vienna: China Tibetology Publishing House; Austrian Academy of Sciences Press, 2015.

Stuart, Daniel M. *S. N. Goenka: Emissary of Insight*. Boston: Shambhala, 2020.

Sujato, Bhikkhu. *A History of Mindfulness: How Insight Worsted Tranquillity in the Satipaṭṭhāna Sutta*. Kerikeri, NZ: Santipada, 2005 [2012].

Sujato, Bhikkhu, trans. *Theragāthā: Verses of the Senior Monks, Pāli-English*. SuttaCentral, 2020 (ebook).

Suzuki, Daisetz Teitarō. *Zen Buddhism: Selected Writings of D. T. Suzuki*. Edited by William Barrett. Garden City, NY: Anchor Doubleday, 1956.

Suzuki, Daisetz Teitarō. "Lectures on Zen Buddhism." In Erich Fromm, ed. *Zen Buddhism and Psychoanalysis*, 1–75. New York: Grove Press, 1960.

Tang, Yi-Yuan., Britta K. Hözel, and Michael I. Posner. "The Neuroscience of Mindfulness Meditation." *Nature Reviews Neuroscience* 16, no. 4 (2015): 213–25.

Taylor, Charles. "Buffered and Porous Selves." *The Immanent Frame: Secularism, Religion, and the Public Sphere*. September 2, 2008. https://tif.ssrc.org/2008/09/02/buffered-and-porous-selves/.

Taylor, Charles. *The Ethics of Authenticity*. Cambridge, MA: Harvard University Press, 1991.

Taylor, Charles. *Modern Social Imaginaries*. Durham: Duke University Press, 2004.

Taylor, Charles. *A Secular Age*. Cambridge, MA: Harvard University Press, 2007.

Taylor, Charles. *Sources of the Self: The Making of Modern Identity*. Cambridge, MA: Harvard University Press, 1989.

Thānissaro Bhikkhu. "Working at Home." Dharmatalks.org. Talks, Writings, and Translations of Thānissaro Bhikkhu, 2008. https://www.dhammatalks.org/mp3_index.html#2008.

Thanissaro Bhikkhu, trans. "Bhikkhu Pāṭimokkha: The Bhikkhus' Code of Discipline." 2007. http://www.accesstoinsight.org/tipitaka/vin/sv/bhikkhu-pati.html. Accessed September 11, 2016.

Thanissaro Bhikkhu, trans "Sallatha Sutta: The Arrow" (SN 36.6). 2013. http://www.accessto insight.org/tipitaka/sn/sn36/sn36.006.than.html. Accessed September 11, 2016.

Thera, Soma. *The Way of Mindfulness: The Satipatthana Sutta and Its Commentary*. 1998 [1941]. http://www.accesstoinsight.org/lib/authors/soma/wayof.html. Accessed October 31, 2016.

Thompson, Evan. "Looping Effects and the Cognitive Science of Mindfulness Meditation." In David McMahan and Erik Braun, eds. *Meditation, Buddhism, and Science*, 47–60. New York: Oxford University Press, 2017.

Thompson, Evan. *Why I Am Not a Buddhist*. New Haven, CT: Yale University Press, 2020.

Thornton, Elizabeth. *The Objective Leader: How to Leverage the Power of Seeing Things as They Are*. New York: St. Martin's Press, 2015.

Trawny, Peter. *Heidegger: A Critical Introduction*. Cambridge: Polity Press, 2019.

Trilling, Lionel. *Sincerity and Authenticity*. Cambridge, MA: Harvard University Press, 1972.

U Pandita, Sayadaw. *Freedom Within: Liberation Teachings on the Satipaṭṭhāna Meditation Practice*. Santa Barbara: Saddhamma Foundation, 2016.

Vaidya, P. L., ed. *Aṣṭasāhastikā Prajñāpāramitā*. Buddhist Sanskrit Texts No. 4. Darbhanga: Mithila Institute, 1960.

Vaidya, P. L., ed. *Gaṇḍavyūha Sūtra*. Buddhist Sanskrit Texts, No. 5. Darbhanga: Mithila Institute, 1960.

Varela, Francisco et al. *The Embodied Mind: Cognitive Science and Human Experience*. Cambridge, MA: MIT Press, 1991.

Varga, Somogy. *Authenticity as an Ethical Ideal*. New York: Routledge, 2011.

Varga, Somogy, and Charles Guignon. "Authenticity." *The Stanford Encyclopedia of Philosophy* (Spring 2020 Edition), Edward N. Zalta (ed.), https://plato.stanford.edu/archives/spr2020/entries/authenticity/.

Verchery, Lina. "The Avatamsaka Sagely Monastery (華嚴聖寺) and New Perspectives on Globalized Buddhism in Canada." In Jason Zuidema, ed. *Understanding the Consecrated Life in Canada: Critical Essays on Contemporary Trends*, 361–76. Waterloo, Ontario: Wilfred Laurier University Press, 2015.

Victoria, Brian Daizen. *Zen at War*. 2nd ed. Lanham, MD: Rowman & Littlefield, 2006.

Vidal, Fernando, and Francisco Ortega. *Being Brains: Making the Cerebral Subject*. New York: Fordham University Press, 2017.

Vipassana Research Institute. *Vipassana, Its Relevance to the Present World: An International Seminar Held at the Indian Institute of Technology, Delhi on 15–17 April 1994*. Igatpuri, India: Vipassana Research Institute, 1995.

Wallace, B. Alan. "Introduction: Buddhism and Science—Breaking Down the Barriers." In B. Alan Wallace, ed. *Buddhism and Science: Breaking New Ground*, 1–29. New York: Columbia University Press, 2003.

Walser, Joseph. "When Did Buddhism Become Anti-Brahmanical? The Case of the Missing Soul." *Journal of the American Academy of Religion* 86, no. 1 (2018): 94–125.

Walshe, Maurice O. *The Long Discourses of the Buddha: A Translation of the Dīgha Nikāya*. Boston: Wisdom Publications, 1995.

Watters, Ethan. *Crazy Like Us: The Globalization of the American Psyche*. New York: Free Press, 2010.

Watts, Alan. *This Is It: and Other Essays on Zen and Spiritual Experience*. New York: Vintage, 1973 [1958].

Westerhoff, Jan. *Nāgārjuna's Madhyamaka: A Philosophical Introduction*. New York and Oxford: Oxford University Press, 2009.

Widdicombe, Lizzie. "The Higher Life: How Mindfulness Became the Road to Success." *New Yorker*. July 6, 2015.

Williams, Paul. *Mahayana Buddhism: The Doctrinal Foundations*. 2nd ed. London and New York: Routledge, 2009.

Wilson, Jeff. *Mindful America: The Mutual Transformation of Buddhist Meditation and American Culture*. New York: Oxford University Press, 2014.

Wittgenstien, Ludwig. *Philosophical Investigations*. New York: MacMillan, 1953.

Wright, Dale. "Introduction: Rethinking Ritual Practice in Zen Buddhism." In Steven Heine and Dale S. Wright, eds. *Zen Ritual: Studies of Zen Theory in Practice*, 3–20. New York: Oxford University Press, 2007.

Wynne, Alexander. *The Origin of Buddhist Meditation*. Routledge Critical Studies in Buddhism. London: Routledge, 2007.

Wynne, Alexander. "Sariputta or Kaccāna? A Preliminary Study of Two Early Buddhist Philosophies of Mind and Meditation." *Journal of the Oxford Centre for Buddhist Studies* 14 (2018): 77–107.

Yancy, George, and Emily McRae. *Buddhism and Whiteness: Critical Reflections*. New York: Lexington Books, 2019.

Yetunde, Pamela Ayo, and Cheryl A. Giles. *Black and Buddhist: What Buddhism Can Teach Us about Race, Resilience, Transformation, and Freedom*. Boston: Shambhala, 2020.

Zigon, Jarrett. "Moral Breakdown and the Ethical Demand: A Theoretical Framework for an Anthropology of Moralities." *Anthropological Theory* 7, no. 2 (2007): 131–50.

Zimmerman, Michael. *A Buddha Within: The Tathāgatagarbhasūtra: The Earliest Exposition of the Buddha-Nature Teaching in India*. Tokyo: The International Research Institute for Advanced Buddhology, Soka University, 2002.

Index

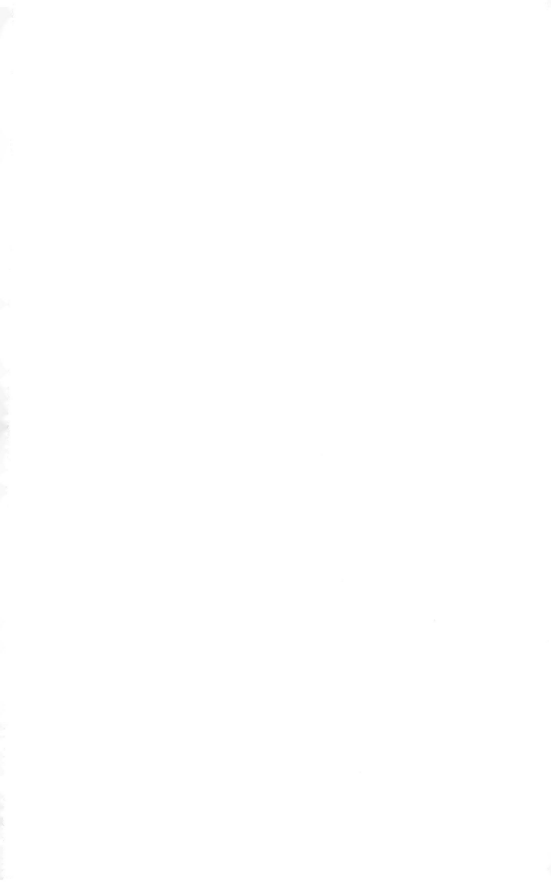